FEEL GOOD

NUTRIGENOMICS

YOUR ROADMAP TO HEALTH

Dr. Amy Yasko

Ph.D., NHD, AMD, HHP, FAAIM

Illustrations and cover art by Melissa Yasko
www.MelissaYasko.com

ISBN 978-0-9915691-0-6

www.DrAmyYasko.com

Occasionally an individual is fortunate enough to have a single supportive person in their lives. I am blessed to be surrounded by loving and supportive people in every aspect of my life. The support that I am given in both my work and home environments gives me the strength and the impetus to spend my time trying to help others to gain optimal health and wellness.

The support I receive gives me the courage to bring forth new ideas. While it may not seem that this should require courage, believe me it does. Many in this universe operate from a position of fear. Fear of the unknown, fear of knowledge, and fear of new ideas. The goal of this book is to bring forth new ideas and to share knowledge.

A very special thank you to Ed, Missie, Jessie and Cassie for giving me the strength, love, courage and confidence to help others.

Contents

Stories of Hope and Health Rewarded

"He who has health, has hope; and he who has hope, has everything." Thomas Carlyle

Your work enlightened me on what I needed to do to regain my health after suffering with chronic migraine and major digestive issues. Your work has made all the difference; a year ago I was in tremendous pain; now I am free.

- Cynthia Albert

We are so thankful for Dr Amy, the countless hours and research she puts in to find all the pieces of the puzzle. As we continue to move forward with Dr Amy's program our son continues to blossom into an amazing young man.

- Cindy Webber, Matthew Webber's Mom

I tried 3 mos of another company's methylation vitamins with little improvement. Your Roadmap supplements have given me my life back. My rheumatologist asked to keep your Roadmap because he had never seen anyone's joints become more stable like mine have since taking your supplements. I am over fifty and shortly after going on your Roadmap my reading vision started improving. My eye doctor scoffed when I said my eyesight was better from my vitamins. Well, her jaw dropped when she tested me and she too asked to keep your Roadmap. She'd never seen anyone's reading eyesight improve like mine! I don't even use readers anymore. Thank you, Dr Amy. Bless you, Dr Amy. My daughter said, "It is good to have our Mom back." Thank you for saving my life.

- Chelsea Winters

Optimizing methylation saved my life!

- Diana Galloway, BSRN

This book, Roadmap to Health, is for anyone who cares about their health. Methyl groups regulate genetic function and are crucial to life itself. With the information provided in this book, you can solve the most complex health problems and unlock anti-aging potential. This book captures Dr. Amy's experience and knowledge about methylation, incorporating her most recent findings. Roadmap is a must read!

- Nancy Mullan, MD

As I look back over the years its truly amazing how much progress has been made and it really is a pleasure to have watched a sick little boy be transformed into a happy and healthy young man! With heart felt gratitude for all the time and expertise you devote to crafting a program that makes such a huge difference in so many lives.

- L. J.

I almost died and suffered tremendously for 5 months before discovering that I have very significant methlyation mutations. No one in the mainstream medical field was able to help me. I had been to 7 emergency rooms and probably about 15 doctors (many "ologists") before discovering your protocol. As soon as I began the ammonia program I noticed a massive shift in a positive direction happening in my body. I finally knew in my heart that I was on the right track and there was finally hope that my suffering would end!! I improved so dramatically and quickly, within the first couple of weeks of starting your protocol, that I was truly shocked and amazed beyond belief. I just wanted to thank you for your research from the bottom of my heart and to thank you for your program because I truly do believe that it is saving my life!! Words cannot express my gratitude! You can use my email and my story however you'd like! I hope to share it with as many people as possible because I want to reach others with similar issues so that maybe it can help them too!!! Having experienced how powerful treating methylation mutations can be, first hand and in such a dramatic way, I'm very passionate about helping to spread the word. Thank you so much again!!

- Katie Sweeney

Dr. Amy Yasko is the hope, the small flickering light, and the quiet in all this chaos of mainstream thoughts on autism...I as a mother of a very special girl am blessed to have crossed paths on the internet and through groups to happen across her breakthrough work...and make other choices for our treatment protocol. ..the lights are on and I'm always home now! Thank you for loving all our children!

- Kari Kane

Dear Dr.Amy, All our thanks goes to you, your family, staff and of course cyber mums! Your tireless work and encouragement is moving us forward and gives us and our brave children a chance to enjoy life and be truly thankful for every single moment we share together, for every new word we hear, for every new achievement that would not be possible without you! We love you Dr.Amy!

- Vesna, Miodrag and Mihail Konstantinova

Federico clinically completely recovered from the autism, we are so grateful to Dr. Amy and her team that they saved Federico's life.

- Debby, Federico and Dalibor

Never say Never to MY boy! This from my boy, the one they told me would probably never talk again, never walk properly again and never be able to hold a pen. Eight years later, I wish those doctors were here to listen to him and to read his stories and to watch him run.

- Jessica James

Dr. Amy's protocol saved my son Andrew, plain and simple. Her brilliant protocol has done absolute miracles for him. A few months before turning 2, Andrew was diagnosed with Autism, and today, the few people I tell about his prior diagnosis are completely shocked, stunned and usually say I didn't know you could fix Autism. Dr. Amy brought him back to me and the words thank you could never suffice.

In March of 2007, my 19 month old son, who had previously been a completely normal child, regressed into Autism. We first tried a biomedical protocol that was not based on individual genetics, and thus it was not tailored to each child's specific needs. Theirs was a try everything on every child and see if it works approach. Not only was this not helpful, due to some specific mutations my son has, some of the amino acid supplements they gave him actually made him so much worse. I then found Dr. Amy's protocol and it made so much sense to test genetics first, and then see what has to be corrected biochemically, specific to Andrew. I didn't know for sure if it was going to work, but her approach seemed to make so much sense.

After being on the protocol for 8 weeks, I had my first glimpses of hope that it could work, as Andrew's seizures slowly started to go away. Then over the next 4 years, little by little, piece by piece, gain by gain Andrew started to come back to me. At 2 years on the program his sensory issues started to get better. At 2 ½ years on the program his expressive and receptive language tested age appropriate and that was truly a milestone. At 3 years on the program, his motor skills greatly improved and he slowly started to become more social again. And at 3 ½ years on the program his articulation tested age appropriate. When he started school for the first time (I had made the decision to keep him out of school for 2 years to focus solely on the protocol) it was at a "normal" school where he did not have any kind of special help. I never told the school of his prior diagnosis and no one ever guessed. Today at 6 ½ years on the protocol Andrew still has a few remaining symptoms like some behavioral issues, inattention and some vestibular problems, but I have great hope the remaining things will go away in time as we continue on. However, with the issues he has remaining, no one would ever guess that 6 ½ years earlier he had been autistic.

- Wendy Moore

Dr. Amy, you have saved our child and family from so many struggles and so much pain. Thankful does not begin to describe our gratitude for your program and how it has changed all of our lives. You have healed our child and so many others. I'm sure as a mom, you know how deep the love for your children goes and how their pain becomes so tightly wound with our own. So, this thanksgiving ... Thank you, Thank you, Thank you ... Thank you for your ground breaking research ... Thank you for your ability to put aside the rest of the world and do what's right ... Thank you for caring so passionately about our children. My son was born in 2005. Never a good sleeper but at 26 months we saw a change, regression and repetitive behavior. 4 weeks later we found out that he had strep and had probably had it since his brother was treated 6 weeks earlier. Not a single "normal" immune reaction EVER, every time he would get sick we would see only neurological changes (OCD, disconnected speech, explosive behavior) Fast forward to Kindergarten ... He was now being treated prophylactic amoxicillin (which kept the neurological symptoms to a point where he could function and remain in school). The explosive behavior continued to be a major issue along with being agitated all the time. Around the holidays that year another mom approached me and said "you do know he can't control that behavior."

She saw inside him, the sweet sensitive little boy, who while punching his teacher was crying out for help. She gave me your book and so began our journey into the Yasko protocol.

He is now in 2nd grade – 21 months into our journey and your program. Attached are pictures from his last field trip. He was relaxed and happy, able to enjoy the day. He is no longer overly stressed and anxious just trying to navigate his world. Last year I had to go on his field trip as support, this year I was able to just go and enjoy him hanging out with his friends. He is reading and comprehending! He is becoming a self-confident learner and person. I had two separate conferences and BOTH teachers independently said the exact same thing "Completely different child from last year, relaxed, happy, gets along with everyone, the ideal student." Yes, that is the same child that punched a teacher this time last year. I just kept pinching myself to make sure it isn't a dream. We have seen these improvements in all aspects of his life. In kindergarten, we coached his soccer team and after the season, concluded that team sports were just too difficult for him. Well, this fall he really wanted to play basketball so we decided to give it a try. He walked into a brand new, very noisy and chaotic gym filled with coaches and teammates he had never met and he stunned us all. He was able to process most of what the coach was telling him, wasn't overly stressed and anxious and most importantly made new friends and "fit in." Can you imagine? He fit in! We could not have possibly dreamed of this day. Oh and on another note – his immune system is starting to function (occasional runny nose, cough and even a recent fever). We are probably only at mile marker 2 of the marathon, but the sheer joy we experience every day, there's no place we'd rather be. The tears have not stopped for us, they started as heartbreaking tears of pure fear and uncertainty of what the future would hold for our son. Trying to take one day at a time and figure out how to be patient with this child and at the same time searching out medical answers. Those tears have turned to tears of sheer joy. The things we will never take for granted. The play date that doesn't have to end promptly at 1 hour while I'm hovering the whole time. The exhausted but happy smile when he gets in the car after school. When he tells ME something's not a big deal. When he brings home a treat for his brothers from school because he can't eat it and is so happy that they can enjoy it and gets the joy from that. But more than anything it's his simple genuine smile. A free and happy smile. Knowing that his future is bright and he is so much stronger because if this journey. He wants to understand every supplement and how it helps his body and brain. And NEVER complains about taking them. And everyone in our family is so much stronger and healthier. I'm so happy we have started the process to health but I see so many children and families struggling every single day. I chose not to think about where we'd be without you. Know you have given us the best and only gift that matters, our child and health.

- Barb Wood Messaros

Forward

This work by Dr. Amy is an example of personalized medicine which connects mainstream biochemistry and genetic roots yet reaches outside the box of conventional medicine. The concept of personalized medicine is a treatment approach which is based on an individual's genetics, and was recommended by the FDA almost a decade ago. This book, *Feel Good Nutrigenomics: Your Roadmap to Health* is an amazing contribution to that concept.

I am a mainstream practicing OB/GYN who found it necessary to look outside of standard medical approaches after our son, Federico was diagnosed with autism not long after his first birthday. As a practicing physician, I attended all possible autism meetings to further educate myself about treatment options. When Federico was 3 years old, I participated in the Autism One national conference in Chicago. I had heard about Dr. Amy and managed to join her talk just as her lecture was starting. The room was packed with doctors and parents with standing room only. I was sitting in the back of the room on the floor leaning up against the wall trying to write some notes. As the lecture progressed I noticed that many people in the room, although very quiet, were not taking notes. I started a conversation with the lady who was sitting next to me on the floor. I asked her "Did Dr. Amy say Methylene or Methyl? "She replied "I do not know and I do not care!" I was surprised. She went on to explain, "I just follow the protocol... I don't worry about mastering the science behind it." She said that she started her daughter on Dr. Amy's protocol a couple of years ago, and she is now healthy and attending a mainstream school. She shared that her family flew to Chicago from Oregon to attend the conference. I asked her why she flew so far to attend the conference if her daughter is doing fine. She tearfully answered "To hug Dr Amy and to thank her in person."

Some of those on the program achieve wonderful results by following the program without delving into the science. As a physician, I am drawn to the scientific basis of the program. At the Q and A session of that same Autism One conference I asked Dr. Amy what type of B12 she would recommend for Federico as I had been advised by Federico's doctor to use B12. Dr. Amy asked me, "Is Federico cystathionine beta synthase homozygote or heterozygote?" I said I did not know. She then asked me "Is he catechol -0 methyl transferase positive?" I did not know. She said, "Then I cannot answer your question, as the type of B12 that I would suggest would depend upon his nutrigenomics." I did not know the answers but I knew for first time in the last 2 years of our struggle with autism that Federico would be just fine. I came home and told my wife Debby that we were switching our plan for him. Since medical school I had maintained my interest in biochemistry and genetics and I knew that Dr. Amy was correct in how to approach Federico's health.

Within 3 months of implementing the protocol, Federico 's hydrogen sulfate and ammonia levels dropped and heavy metals started pouring out of his little body. This was correlating with his rapid clinical improvement. Federico graduated from the school for autistic kids at age 4. As Federico smoothly transitioned into mainstream education, Debby wanted to continue speech, occupational, and behavioral therapies as surveillance, but was told that he no longer needed it. Federico's English became crystal clear and he began mimicking my Czech accent for fun, which was hilarious. Federico is now 7 1/2 years old and is a star in the 2nd grade. His charming and very social personality is loved by his classmates and teachers alike. He enjoys playing piano, sports, drama class, play dates, and learning Spanish. People do not believe that he was ever diagnosed as autistic. Having said that, Federico continues nutritional supplementation, and has inspired many "healthy" members of our family to embark on Dr. Amy's program. Her program is not just about autism. And the premise of this book is that all of us need to be thinking about nutrigenomics when it comes to our health.

Despite the fact that I am member of several national scientific societies of mainstream conservative orientation, I still believe that my mom, Federico's grandmother, sent us Dr. Amy from heaven to save our Federico. I am pleased that she has written a book to bring the concepts that helped Federico to many more people, with the intention of helping them with this program for health based on nutrigenomics.

Dr. Dalibor Hradek

First recipient OBHG Physician of the Year Award, 2014

CHAPTER 1

Why a Roadmap

Changing the way you look at your health creates an open road in front of you, poised for a healthier life. Once you recognize that you actually do have control over your own health and wellness, you can then chart that journey. Looking at where you are today and where you want to be in the future defines the road you need to take. For some who are already vibrant and healthy it is a short trip, for others it may be the marathon I have been helping people traverse since starting my private practice well over a decade ago. Regardless if you are merely looking to support an already healthy lifestyle or to change years of deteriorating health, this shift in approach enables you to have control in a way you most likely have never imagined.

I began using this approach with adults who had issues with Chronic Fatigue, ALS, MS, IBS and Parkinson's disease. I had spent years studying biochemical and molecular pathways for my undergraduate degree in chemistry, PhD in Microbiology/ Immunology and my fellowships in Pediatric Immunology, Cancer Research, Cell Biology as well as working to design molecular tests and products for pharmaceutical and biotechnology companies. I found that I think in biochemical pathways. The way some people have an innate sense of direction I see pathways in the body. I have literally gotten lost driving my own children home from school, yet I can tell you how different natural products join together in traffic circles in your body.

When I moved from a metropolitan area to rural Maine, I not only moved demographically. I also shifted scientifically from considering the impact of pharmaceutical products on the pathways in our system, to thinking about the use of natural products to achieve similar results; how herbs and supplements could have a positive impact on those very same biochemical and molecular pathways.

In my private practice, I used natural products to have a positive effect on biochemical and molecular pathways in the body, finding that was what was helping to improve health for adults with a range of chronic inflammatory conditions. One day a woman I was working with asked for my help with her young daughter's inflammatory gut condition. The use of herbs and other natural supplements not only helped the gut but also helped to restore her verbal language. Unbeknown to me, this young girl was autistic. I am embarrassed to admit but I was not fully aware of autism at that time. This was 1999 and my focus for almost twenty years had been medical, pharmaceutical and biotechnology approaches to solve standard research topics in a more traditional arena. My more recent foray into herbs and natural supplements, along with courses in natural health care had only begun in 1998. While I was thrilled with the ability to use natural products to impact known biochemical and molecular pathways in the body, the success with respect to adult inflammatory conditions was satisfying but not a surprise. The well documented impact of herbs on inflammatory conditions along with a focus on limiting over excitation of nerves lent itself to these health imbalances. But autism, that was something that had been outside of my radar, it was not a field being approached at that time via biochemical and molecular researchers and the finding that I had helped to restore language in this young girl by working to address inflammation in her gut was totally unexpected. At that time, there were very few language therapists in Maine. The same therapist working in the rural mountains of western Maine was also responsible for language therapy in the 'big city' of Portland, Maine. And so via speech therapists, word of the success of this program spread from person to person in Maine.

At the time of this entree into the autism community I was still firmly rooted in adult inflammatory conditions coupled with a strong emphasis on the role of spirituality in health. It was the 4th of July weekend, 2002, and I had literally just finished giving a talk to a group of monks in a friary in Yonkers, NY about the role of spirituality in health when my office in Maine called about the outpouring of requests from mothers of children with autism. The internet is a wonderful tool, and word had spread beyond Maine to the *real* big city, New York City, citing the ability of this program to help those with autism. It was a learning curve for me personally to truly understand autism, just as it was a learning curve for anyone choosing to use this program.

From the onset **I have always believed in sharing the rationale behind choices of herbs and supplements; giving the power and control to each individual to make informed personal health care choices.** What this means is that there is a steep learning curve to be able to make decisions governing your own or your child's health. I have spent the past decade pouring my heart and soul into autism and refining the program, generating more resources to help understand and implement the program, and now have come full circle to include adults with inflammatory conditions, those simply looking for a healthier lifestyle, as well as those with autism on this journey to better health and wellness.

This program began with adults, was adapted to help those with autism, and in this book I now define the steps to take to chart your own Roadmap to health. **This is not just about autism; it is about health and well-being.** I believe that autism, as with other chronic conditions is a multifactorial condition. That underlying genetic susceptibility, along with exposure to infectious agents, toxic chemical and the stress of lifestyle all contribute to complex health issues. In this book I will make analogies using the concept of a Roadmap to help you to visualize the contribution of genetics, epigenetics, as well as other factors that play a role in health. Understanding the contributing factors gives you the information needed to pick the right tools to get back on a path to health and well-being. Every child with autism has a parent, a grandparent and siblings, and hopefully will have children of their own someday. The predisposing genetics come from somewhere. According to current statistics the rate of autism is one in fifty. In other words, with a rate of 1 in 50, every one of us has a relative, a child, an uncle a cousin or a brother that may be on the autism spectrum. Even if those same related genetics are not manifesting as autism they may be a factor in Parkinson's, CFS, MS, Lupus or some other inflammatory condition. **Recognizing that this is not just about autism, and realizing that the genetics are inherited in a familial pattern, means every single person in today's society needs to be thinking about charting their personal Roadmap to health.**

Alzheimer's disease, Chronic Fatigue syndrome, ADD/ADHD as well as autism are increasing at an alarming rate. While medicine has made incredible strides clearly we need to think about a different approach to deal with a range of chronic health conditions in today's society.   What I have been sharing is a paradigm shift in how we deal with chronic conditions**. The idea is to make you the expert on your own path to health.** I share the information to give you the tools to make informed decisions in conjunction with your own doctor/practitioner.

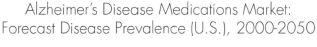

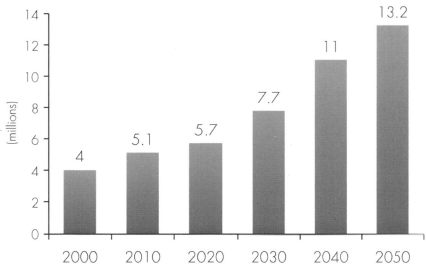

Alzheimer's Disease Medications Market:
Forecast Disease Prevalence (U.S.), 2000-2050

The number of Alzheimer's Disease patients is expected
to more than triple over the next 50 years

Source: Frost & Sullivan

When the increase in Alzheimer's was first noted the explanation was that people are living longer so of course more of them are dying of Alzheimer's disease. Today, Alzheimer's is listed as one of the leading causes of death in this country.

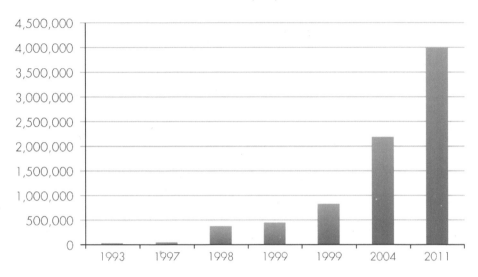

Estimated number of people with
CFS in U.S. population

When the number of individuals with CFS was on the rise, the explanation was that the stress of women working while raising their children was to blame.

The increase in ADD/ADHD was cited as being due to poor health choices for children's snacks and too many families with two working parents. By 1997, the number of children labeled as having "ADHD" had risen alarmingly to 4.4 million and by 2009 the figure was closer to six million, with approximately one in every 10 children now diagnosed with the disorder.

1987
(Diagnostic and Statistical Manual of Mental Disorders III-R. Published by the American Psychiatric Association Washington, DC. 1987)

0

1988
(CHADD, http://www.cchrint.org /psycho-pharmaceutical-front-groups/chadd/#_edn10

500,000

1999
(Report of the U.S. Surgeon General on Mental Health)

1,900,000
Avg (1,400,000 to 2,300,000)

2003
(CDC: MMRW 9/2/03)

4,200,000

2008
(Vital and Health Statistics Report from CDC's National Center for Health Statistics - July 2008)

4,500,000

2009
(Block, 2009)

6,000,000

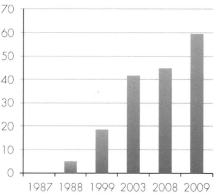

Studies of ADHD Prevalence (per 100,000)

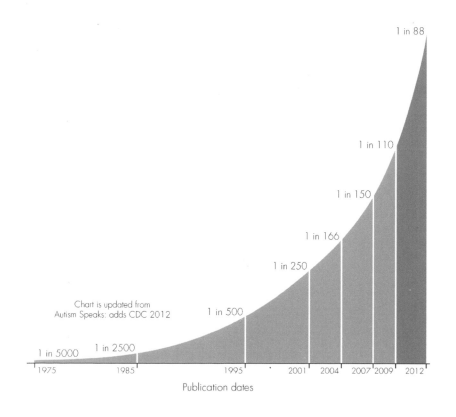

Chart is updated from Autism Speaks: adds CDC 2012

Publication dates

"In 2002 the Center for Disease Control estimated that autism affected about 1 in 150 children. By 2012 the CDC estimate had increased to 1 in 88. Now, according to the latest revision of the estimate recently released, autism affects 1 in 50 children. That's a phenomenal 300 percent increase in 11 years" (National Health Statistics, March 2013). **This alarming increase in autism has been explained by better diagnosis.**

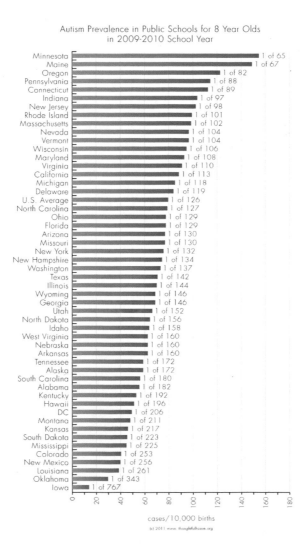

Autism Prevalence in Public Schools for 8 Year Olds
in 2009-2010 School Year

Minnesota	1 of 65
Maine	1 of 67
Oregon	1 of 82
Pennsylvania	1 of 88
Connecticut	1 of 89
Indiana	1 of 97
New Jersey	1 of 98
Rhode Island	1 of 101
Massachusetts	1 of 102
Nevada	1 of 104
Vermont	1 of 104
Wisconsin	1 of 106
Maryland	1 of 108
Virginia	1 of 110
California	1 of 113
Michigan	1 of 118
Delaware	1 of 119
U.S. Average	1 of 126
North Carolina	1 of 127
Ohio	1 of 129
Florida	1 of 129
Arizona	1 of 130
Missouri	1 of 130
New York	1 of 132
New Hampshire	1 of 134
Washington	1 of 137
Texas	1 of 142
Illinois	1 of 144
Wyoming	1 of 146
Georgia	1 of 146
Utah	1 of 152
North Dakota	1 of 156
Idaho	1 of 158
West Virginia	1 of 160
Nebraska	1 of 160
Arkansas	1 of 160
Tennessee	1 of 172
Alaska	1 of 172
South Carolina	1 of 180
Alabama	1 of 182
Kentucky	1 of 192
Hawaii	1 of 196
DC	1 of 206
Montana	1 of 211
Kansas	1 of 217
South Dakota	1 of 223
Mississippi	1 of 225
Colorado	1 of 253
New Mexico	1 of 256
Louisiana	1 of 261
Oklahoma	1 of 343
Iowa	1 of 767

cases/10,000 births

(c) 2011 www.thoughtfulhouse.org

I see these as excuses, not as explanations.

I feel that we live in a society where we are stressed emotionally, financially, physically and exposed to a range of toxins in our environment. Combining underlying genetic susceptibility with these other factors creates all the ingredients for a perfect storm By understanding where our weak points are located, where the 'accidents' are on our particular highway of life, it is possible to bypass those detours, accidents and breakdowns and chart a better Roadmap to Health. *This* is the approach that I used in my private practice for adults, for children and have been sharing online at no cost. This is the approach that is explored through this book, simplified by analogies of driving a car and following a Roadmap that we can all understand. *This* is the approach that will help you and your doctor to bring you better health and well-being.

State-based Prevalence Data of ADHD Diagnosis Percent of Youth 4-17 ever diagnosed with Attention-Deficit/Hyperactivity Disorder: National Survey of Children's Health, 2007

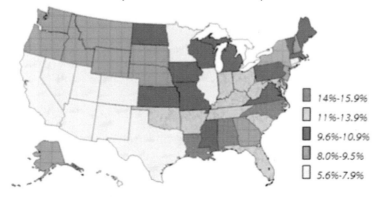

14%-15.9%
11%-13.9%
9.6%-10.9%
8.0%-9.5%
5.6%-7.9%

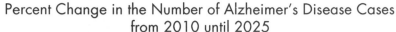

Percent Change in the Number of Alzheimer's Disease Cases
from 2010 until 2025

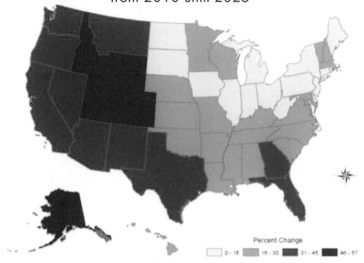

Just as with a Roadmap and a car you can travel anywhere in this country, so too does the impact of chronic health issues traverse the country. While the incidence of ADHD, Alzheimer's CFS or autism may differ depending on where you live, there is no state in this country that is free from these chronic health conditions. This is why a program to help you to take charge of your heath, regardless of your physical location is so relevant in today's society.

This program helps you to understand a central pathway in your body, a pathway that is directly related to a range of health conditions, a pathway that in my opinion is *the* key pathway to life and health. I personally believe that if this pathway cannot function, or is severely compromised that it is inconsistent with the ability to survive. That is how important I feel the **Methylation**

Cycle is for your health, the health of your children, your grandchildren, your parents and grandparents.

This pathway is so important that I truly believe that everyone should have an equal ability to understand it and to make informed choices to support it in their body. The overriding tenant of this program is to give you the tools you need to make informed personalized decisions about your own health.   The more information you have, the more power and control you have. No one is going to be more interested in your health and wellness than you are. No matter how lovely, smart and involved your doctor is, with the volume of patients he/she has to see each day there is no way they can give you the level of priority that you can give yourself. This is not to say that you can do this solely on your own, without your doctor. I am not suggesting that at all. What I am suggesting is a paradigm shift in how we view healthcare. Instead of the classic view of the doctor in the white coat dispensing medicine and answers where you obediently take whatever is given with no explanation, this program gives you the tools to change that dynamic and take charge of your own health by understanding the role, importance and genetics of the critical **Methylation Cycle** in the body.

CHAPTER 2

New Approaches for the Challenges of Today's Society

Once upon a time... life was a lot simpler. On the heels of the Second World War, the 1950's was a time of renewed hope and innocence. When men wore grey flannel suits and women wore dresses with pinched waists and high heels. Years ago, in most families mom stayed at home and dad went to work.   "The Donna Reed" show played on black and white televisions.   TV was first becoming a dominant mass media phenomenon and the UNIVAC computer, taking up 943 cubic feet of space became the first commercial computer to attract widespread public attention. It was at this time, in the middle of the twentieth century, that optimism was high for eradicating disease. The first antibiotics were developed in the 1950's and the distribution of the polio vaccine began in 1955. The medical community felt that they had the tools to deal with infectious diseases. Serious bacterial infections could be handled by antibiotics such as penicillin, streptomycin and other new antibiotics on the frontier.

Viral epidemics would be prevented by vaccinations. And the world would be safe from infectious disease.

In contrast, today's society is more complex and so are our health issues. There were 40 million cars on the road in 1950, compared with over a billion cars worldwide last year with estimates that the number will double to close to 2 billion by 2035. That is an incredible increase in vehicles along with an equivalent increase in carbon monoxide, nitrogen dioxide, sulfur dioxide, benzene, formaldehyde, and polycyclic hydrocarbons from the exhaust of these vehicles.

Our environment has changed drastically since the 1950's. With the industrialization of the world, the amounts of toxic metals have increased markedly. In today's society, levels of lead, mercury and cadmium are all found to be in far greater concentrations than what is recommended for optimal health and longevity. These heavy metals are contributing to the epidemic of degenerative disease we are seeing today in every country in all age groups.

"Heavy metals are present in our air, drinking water, food, and countless human-made chemicals and products. They are taken into the body via inhalation, ingestions, and skin absorption. If heavy metals enter and accumulate in body tissues faster than the body's detoxification pathways can dispose of them, a gradual

buildup of these toxins will occur. High-concentration exposure is not necessary to produce a state of toxicity in the body, as heavy metals accumulate in body tissues and, over time, can reach toxic concentration levels. Human exposure to heavy metals has risen dramatically in the last 50 years as a result of an exponential increase in the use of heavy metals in industrial processes and products. Today, chronic exposure comes from mercury-amalgam dental fillings, lead-based paint, tap water, chemical residues in processed foods, and personal care products-cosmetics, shampoo and other hair products, mouthwash, toothpaste and soap. In today's industrial society, there is no escaping exposure to toxic chemicals and metals. In addition to the hazards both at home and outdoors, many occupations involve daily metal exposure. Over 50 professions entail exposure to mercury alone. These include physicians, pharmaceutical workers, any dental occupation, laboratory workers, hairdressers, painters, welders, metalworkers, battery makers, engravers, photographers, visual artists, and potters" (Pouls, M., Extreme Health, Univ. Michigan).

Toxic metals accumulate in our bodies over our lifetimes, beginning with the amounts we receive from our mothers during pregnancy; metals we are inoculated with during vaccination; and the metals we consume and breathe every day thereafter. It is clear to see that health approaches that were based on a society that existed in the 1950's are outdated in terms of the needs of today's environmental milieu.

Fifty years ago we did not have the stress of two working parents in almost every household. The divorce rate has doubled since the 1950s, with more of us living in single parent households. Serving the role of both mom and dad creates additional stress. We have fast food, fast cars, and a fast pace of life with all the stressors that go with it. And all of that was before September 11, 2001. Now we have fears of terrorism in our own backyards to compound these other tensions in our lives.

The mid twentieth century saw the advent of antibiotics. While these medical treatments were successful for acute bacterial illness, those methods are not well suited for the prevalent chronic inflammatory conditions we encounter in the twenty first century. However, for the most part, our approach to infectious agents has not changed drastically from that time. *"Medicine's molecular revolution is long overdue. By now, enthusiasts led us to believe, gene therapy and related treatments should have transformed clinical practice. Diseases, they told us, would be cured at their genetic roots, by repairing defective DNA or by disabling the genes of infectious microbes. But it has proved frustratingly difficult to make these methods work in the clinic, if you get sick, your doctor will probably still treat you with the pills and potions of old fashioned medicinal chemistry"* (Check, E. Nature).

It has reached a point where it is not sufficient to merely take a drug for an illness. At one time it was enough to take an antibiotic to treat a bacterial infection. That is no longer the case. The entire picture with respect to disease is not as straightforward as it once was.

We can attempt to lower the stress in our lives. However, for many of us the stress in our lives is a given, not a variable. While we may be able to affect <u>how</u> we react to the stress, we are unable to lower the total burden of stress that we are under. We can try to reduce our personal toxin burden, and our exposure to infectious diseases. Yet, unless we become like the "boy in the bubble" and isolate ourselves from our environment this becomes virtually impossible. We can eat organic foods, use only natural materials in our homes, use cleansers without chemicals, and eat chemical free foods, and drink filtered water. All of this adds another layer of complication and stress to our already overburdened lives. We still need to go out and interact in the world where everyone else <u>does not</u> create a chemical free, toxin free, microbe free environment. We can however do our best in each of these categories. **If we can make even a small difference in each category of these risk factors, then we can reduce the likelihood of having chronic health conditions.**

Clearly, a number of factors contribute and interact to create the ultimate scenario of nonideal health. The more stressed your system and the greater your metal and toxic burden, the more likely you are to be harboring infectious organisms like bacteria, viruses and yeast. The number of infectious pathogens to which an individual has been exposed (infectious burden) has been correlated with a number of conditions, including coronary artery disease, gastric ulcers, and cervical cancer just to name a few. The proven and suspected roles of microbes is not limited to physical ailments; infections are increasingly being examined as associated causes of or possible contributors to a variety of serious, chronic neuropsychiatric disorders and to developmental problems, especially in children (Institute of Medicine Report, Natl. Academies Press).

"The problem with diabetes, hypertension, heart disease and other common ailments is untangling the genetic factors from a person's lifestyle and environment. What causes an individual's diabetes, overeating or bad genes? Human habits make it more challenging. Genetics certainly isn't the only factor in diseases. A hundred years ago, diabetes was much less of a problem, and in the last century human genes haven't changed much. What has changed, however, are eating habits and physical activity" (Berger, E. Houston Chronicle).

An extension of these concepts is that most health conditions that we see today will in fact be multifactorial in nature. While we cannot change your genetic susceptibility, **we can look at your genetic profile and use nutritional supplementation to help to bypass underlying genetic weaknesses to lower your genetic risk factors. This will help you to achieve optimal health when used in conjunction with a program to reduce some of the other risk factors such as environmental toxins and infectious agents.**

Although the genetics we inherit may not have changed since the 1950's the collective impact of the other risk factors for nonideal health have increased. **By reducing the role of underlying predisposing genetics it can help to tip the scale back in the balance of better health**. The goals of this protocol are to

- reduce the impact of underlying nutrigenomic mutations
- reduce the impact of compounds that overexcite your nerves
- and to improve the environment in your system in terms of microbes and toxins

While the concept of genetics, and toxins and viruses and bacteria may seem overwhelming, this is a program you can understand and master. A Roadmap, which is something we all understand, can be seen as an analogy to the pathways in our body. Visualizing the path to health as a road we traverse in life is a familiar and comfortable concept that allows you to conquer and have control over your own health.

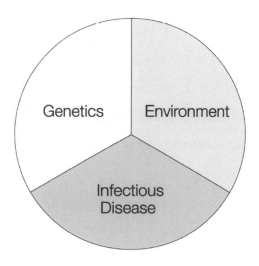

CHAPTER 3

Defining a New Path

Years ago the lead time for my private appointment schedule had stretched to five years. I mention this not to be all about me, because **I truly believe that real healthcare is actually all about you.** I mention the extent of the waiting list as evidence that the program that I use really does make a positive difference. In response to the length of that waiting list I no longer offer personal consults of any type. Instead, all of the resources to implement this program are shared online at no charge. This allows equal access to this program and enables you to implement it in conjunction with your own doctor in a timeframe that works for you.

In today's society of social media, word spreads rapidly, and it was that positive feedback that allowed for my small private practice in a rural town in the mountains of Maine to grow to literally a worldwide client base of over thousands of individuals. At that time I did not, and I still do not feel that anyone should have to wait five years to get on the path to better health. I made a paradigm shift; I stopped offering private appointments and started sharing all of my information online at no charge. With this approach everyone would have access to it and could implement it to the extent they wanted with their own doctor. This was the only way I could think of to be fair to everyone. If I were to continue with private appointments how would I pick whom to work with? The parent with the child most severely affected with autism? The parent of multiple affected children on the spectrum? The adult with the most health problems who still needs to deal with an ailing husband and a mother with dementia while caring for her four children? There was no way to pick, all of you need and deserve equal time, help and attention. So that is why **the answer was simply to share**. To share all the details and resources on line at no charge and ask that all you do is to take advantage of those resources to have the tools to help yourself.

This paradigm shift in approaching health by simply sharing all of the resources online at no cost always causes me to think of a quote from one of my favorite poems, The Invitation by Oriah Mountain Dreamer. *"It doesn't interest me to know where you live or how much money you have. I want to know if you can get up after the night of grief and despair, weary and bruised to the bone and do what needs to be done to feed the children."* It is not about picking the individual to work with who is willing to pay the most for your time, or the one who screams the loudest that they need the help, it is about helping anyone who is willing to get up bruised and weary and still do what needs to be done for their families.

The other piece I ask is to find a doctor or practitioner you can work with that will help you to implement the program. Since I do not charge for my time and resources I feel that you can instead spend the funds on an appointment with the doctor/practitioner of your choice. I would encourage you to ask others on the chat group (www.ch3nutrigenomics.com) about their choices of physicians. At each of my conferences there are a number of doctors/practitioners who attend and are familiar with the program. There is a lovely array of doctors, male and female, young and old with a range of different personalities and medical backgrounds who have attended the conferences and may be the right fit for you. I do not suggest or give out names, I leave that to others so that you can get an honest unfiltered opinion from individuals who are actually using the program and will let you know what they think. Remember though, this program is designed for *you* to take advantage of the resources to understand the program yourself and not just to rely on your doctor to tell you what to do. This idea is that **knowledge is power** and the more you know the better you can work with your doctor/practitioner for true and lasting good health.

In the past you went to your physician who was the source of all greater knowledge in a long white coat who told you what to do and what to take and you trusted that he or she had all of the answers, you obediently followed that advice without having to think. There is nothing wrong with that approach. It's just that I do it differently. I share all of the "why' behind the suggestions. I donate my time essentially 24/7 to share this information and then the expectation is that those who choose to follow the program are willing to put in *their* time to understand the "why" so they can make informed choices, which they then share with their own doctor/practitioner and in many cases actually serve to educate their own physicians. I understand that not everyone is comfortable with this approach and that is okay too. I have found that I can help more people and pay it forward by sharing information and giving others the opportunity to "**read it, learn it, live it**".

At this time I do continue to make personal comments on tests that are ordered through Holistic Health International (www.holistichealth.com) for those who still want my personal feedback that they can then share with their own doctors. However, the majority of those who follow this program do not run tests for my comments but do the entire program via testing through their own doctor. We have over 56,000 people on the Facebook page following the program and about 15,000 on the chat group; only a small fraction of these individuals find it necessary to have my comments on tests. The majority of those using this program do so entirely by taking advantage of the tools online at no cost to educate themselves and then work to implement the program with their own doctor/practitioner. My role is to provide you with the tools you need to understand the program and then to connect you with others on the program so that you can make informed choices regarding a choice of health care providers as well as your own health care regime.

The workbook, DVDs, PPTs, transcripts of the content of all talks and the chat group are all online for everyone at no cost. The chat group has thousands of posts that I have written answering questions about the program. I do not have appointments and I also do not charge for my time. I work seven days a week, donating my time to help to answer questions and to comment on tests run through HHI. What I ask from anyone using the program is that you take advantage of these resources so you understand the program and can share your knowledge with your own doctor for implementation of the program. My feeling is that I am willing to donate my time to help all of you, and what I need from each of you is to take the time to use the resources so you have an understating of the information that I work so hard to share with all of you. Yes, this is a major paradigm shift in how we view health and wellness. **It means you have power and** control over your own health, but it also means you have to take some responsibility and initiative in terms of making the time to read it, learn it and live it.

CHAPTER 4

Driving the Car

I have no sense of direction in a car. I have literally gotten lost driving my children home from school on a route I have traveled daily because I was distracted. Just because I have driven on a highway from point A to point B before is no guarantee that I can traverse that path again without getting horrendously lost. Yet, I can navigate in biochemical pathways. I see the movement of amino acids and signaling pathways for genes the way some people have an innate directional sense in a car. What this book will do is help you to see how **biochemical pathways in the body are as easy to navigate as roadways with your car**. This program breaks down the complexities of biochemistry and molecular biology to a series of traffic circles and detours and dead ends. **If you have learned to drive a car, you can learn to take control over your own health choices.** While it may seem overwhelming at the start it is no different than the feeling of being overwhelmed the first time you drove a 3000 pound motor vehicle.

The sheer responsibility of driving a car that weighs over a ton is daunting. You get behind the wheel and you realize that if you are not careful, if you don't know the rules of the road, if you lose concentration that you can actually kill someone or kill yourself. Driving a car is no small responsibility yet we all learn to do it, and it becomes second nature for us. I recall the first time I sat in a car for drivers education. There were so many things to worry about simultaneously, the side view mirrors, the rear view mirror, looking ahead over the hood for what was in front, trying to remember which was the gas and which was the brake pedal, using the blinkers trying not to speed and of course what to do at a four way intersection without traffic lights. Overwhelming at first, yet over time it became commonplace and eventually driving becomes something we do without consciously thinking about it.

Learning to navigate this program may initially seem overwhelming. But as the many individuals who have been using it for years will tell you, it becomes a way of life, second nature over time. The veterans of this program serve as the moderators on the discussion group. All of the questions I have answered about the program are archived and searchable on the discussion group. The workbook with details for implementing the program is also available online no charge. The PPTs, the DVDs, the transcripts of the talks are also available online at no charge. Once you have a greater understanding of the process you are then in the position to share your choices with your own doctor/practitioner, and have your doctor help you to implement the program. This keeps your doctor in the loop, yet gives you control over your own natural health choices. I truly believe that knowledge is power. **The more you know, the less scary health choices become, and the more power you have over your own healthcare.**

CHAPTER 5

Nutrigenomics

The long-term goal of molecular medicine, as well as molecular nutrition/nutrigenomics, is to have personalized healthcare that takes into account an individual's genetic, environmental and infectious disease profile. The combination of components that interact to cause multifactorial health problems may be different in every individual. There may be slight or enormous changes in the relative contributions of each of these components to disease. Personalized medicine enables your cells to get the specific support they require to be balanced. *"individualized healthcare, once a seemingly utopian fantasy, is steadily gaining ground as a rational approach…"* (Nature Medicine).

The field of **nutrigenomics** is the study of how natural products and supplements can interact with particular genes to decrease the risk of diseases. By looking at an individual's particular DNA in these nutritional pathways it enables one to make supplement choices based on personalized genetics, rather than using the same support for every individual regardless of their unique needs. With knowledge of imbalances in nutritional genetic pathways it is possible to utilize combinations of nutrients, foods and natural nucleotides to bypass mutations and restore proper pathway function.

Nutrigenomics integrates concepts in molecular biology and genomics to study the ability of foods and nutritional supplements to interact with genes to influence our health and lower the genetic risk component for multifactorial disease. This field of nutrigenomics is perhaps best described by the group that is dedicated to promoting this new science of nutritional genomics. According to the National Center of Excellence in Nutritional Genomics at UC Davis, *"The science of nutrigenomics seeks to provide a molecular understanding for how common dietary chemicals (i.e., nutrition) affect health by altering the expression and/or structure of an individual's genetic makeup. Just as pharmacogenomics has led to the concept of "personalized medicine" and "designer drugs", so will the new field of nutrigenomics open the way for "personalized nutrition." In other words, by understanding our nutritional needs, our nutritional status, and our genotype, nutrigenomics should enable individuals to manage better their health and well-being by precisely matching their diets with their unique genetic makeup."*

The nutrigenomic results that I analyze in my protocol focus on genetic weaknesses in a particular pathway that I call the *Methylation Cycle*. (This analysis is available at no cost at www.knowyourgenetics.com.) This central pathway in the body is particularly amenable to nutrigenomic screening for genetic weaknesses. Defects in this cycle lay the appropriate groundwork for the further assault of environmental and infectious agents and can result in an increased risk for additional health conditions including diabetes, cardiovascular disease, thyroid dysfunction, neurological inflammation, chronic viral infection, neurotransmitter imbalances, atherosclerosis, cancer, aging, neural tube defects, Alzheimer's disease and autism.

By looking at diagrammatic representations of the Methylation Cycle and relating the effects of genetic polymorphisms to biochemical pathways, we are able to draw a personalized map for each individual's imbalances which may impact upon their health. By identifying the precise areas of genetic fragility, it is then possible to target appropriate nutritional supplementation of these pathways to optimize the functioning of these crucial biochemical processes.

Brief overview of potential consequences of variations in the genes in the methylation pathway including:

Increased Homocysteine

- Renal Failure
- Stroke
- Heart Attack
- Diabetes
- Alzheimer's disease
- Neural defects

Decreased Methylation

- Cancer
- Aging
- Cardiovascular disease
- Neurological issues
- Retroviral transmission
- Neural defects
- Down's syndrome

Decreased BH4

- Diabetes
- Atypical phenylketonuria (PKU)
- Decreased dopamine levels
- Decreased serotonin levels
- Hypertension
- Atherosclerosis
- Decreased NOS
- Endothelial dysfunction

Elevated Ammonia

- Flapping tremors of extended arms
- Disorientation, brain fog
- Hyperactive reflexes
- Activation of NMDA receptors leading to glutamate excitotoxicity
- Tremor of the hands
- Paranoia, panic attacks
- Memory loss
- Hyperventilation (often associated with decreased CO2)
- CNS toxicity
- Alzheimer's disease

Four basic steps have been defined as working to deduce information in our genes to developing personalized healthcare. These steps include, "

- *Defining the functional elements of the human genome,*
- *determining which genes or pathways are altered in a disease state,*
- *discovering inherited sequence patterns contributing to disease,*
- *applying genomics information to improve clinical practices"* (Wills, R. Modern Drug Discovery).

Molecular medicine will eventually be able to use sophisticated drugs that are concerned with precise mechanisms of action to accomplish this task. *"We're saying if we know what changes in genetic make-up drive a particular disease, then we can design a drug tailored for the individual requirements of that patient"* (Burke, M., BioPeople). Improved diagnostics permit better drug dosing to identify the percentage of patients that will respond to customized treatments. *"Though the cost and logistics of implementing individualized therapy may appear to be prohibitive...the value of targeted therapy ...and the appeal of customized therapy is evident"* (Nature Medicine). This is underscored by the recent finding that only patients with a certain genetic makeup gain any benefit from particular commonly prescribed drugs. The study helps to support the concept of personalized medicine, the choice of drugs that work best for an individual patient based on genetic testing (Chasman, D., JAMA).

Nutrigenomics uses natural products to affect cellular and molecular processes. *"Most of chronic diseases are related to cellular alterations which can, in part, be influenced by nutrients. Similarly, the efficiency of therapeutic drugs can be modulated by nutrients"* (International Society for Molecular Nutrition and Therapy).

Both disciplines, molecular medicine as well as nutrigenomics, take advantage of the strides made in the Human Genome Project that allow us to utilize simple genetic tests to look at our genetic weaknesses.

The goal of the Human Genome Project was to identify all the approximately 25,000 genes in human DNA and to determine the sequences or "spelling" of the 3 billion chemical base pairs that make up human DNA. This project was completed in June of 2000.

As a direct consequence of having the complete sequence of the human genome, research has focused on identifying particular genes that are involved with specific diseases. The challenge is to identify disease causing genes and clarify their roles. *"The advent of microarray technology has accelerated the pace of gene expression analysis, allowing the simultaneous analysis of thousands of genes"* (Salowsky, R., BioPharm International).

While the first step that emerged from the Human Genome Project has been to identify genes associated with a particular disease, the next step is to use this information to look for the presence of these genes in an individual person. Rather than looking at complete gene profiles it is also possible to look at particular changes in the "spelling" of your DNA in only specific areas of interest. In this way, you can more quickly get a sense of known genetic weaknesses. Companies that offer this service enable you to look at twenty or so genes of interest that may affect your susceptibility to heart disease, inflammation, detoxification or simply your ability to absorb nutrients.

In order to find relationships between genetic changes and the susceptibility to disease this testing is done utilizing single nucleotide polymorphisms otherwise known as SNP's (pronounced *snips*). This process systematically compares genomes of those individuals with a disease or a known health condition to the corresponding DNA of a healthy population. To identify a SNP is a very arduous and time consuming process, as there may be 400 or more genes in a shared region making it difficult to identify changes and trends. However, once it has been identified, making practical use of this information is quick and straightforward. Small differences in these SNPs not only reflect susceptibility to disease but may also affect how people respond to drugs (Abbott, A. Nature).   These new genetic testing systems will enable the testing of a patient's genes before prescribing any drug.   Thus, the doctor will know in advance if a drug is potentially lethal or ineffective for them.

As recently as ten years ago, this technology was only a vision in the future *"the new tissue samples that patients can submit on their own, as from a swab from their cheek, are not yet ready to allow us to totally profile out nutrient needs"* (Check, E., Nature). Yet today, this ability exists to personalize nutrition based programs that are based on our individual nutrigenomic profiling.

CHAPTER 6

Your Personal Vehicle

For the purposes of your Roadmap to health, one way we can look at your DNA that you inherit at birth is a car you are given that needs to last your entire lifetime. This car allows you to travel on your personal journey through life. It is this car and knowledge of its mechanical issues that enable us to chart your personal Roadmap to health. Some people may be more fortunate in the quality of the car they receive; they may receive cars that are designed to last two hundred thousand miles without needing much more than a simple tune up. Others may receive a vehicle that has significant issues. If we know what those mechanical issues are, we can take care of that car so that its problems can be bypassed for a smoother ride through life. What we are given is what we need to contend with. We have very little control over the DNA that we inherit. The car we get is what we are saddled with for our entire lives.

In order to get an understanding of the impact of genetics, it is important that you fully realize that the DNA you have inherited will not change. This is the DNA you will have for your entire lifetime. The same DNA you have at birth is the DNA that you have in the later years of your life. Virtually every cell in your body contains identical DNA, which is why blood, saliva, hair, fingernails can be used to evaluate your personal DNA. There are approximately 25,000 genes in the human body that code for proteins, but it is not practical to look at all 25,000 genes. While every cell in the body essentially contains the information about your total genetic profile, tests that look at genetics choose *specific genes* to evaluate and look for changes or mutations.

I personally believe in only looking for changes in the DNA in well-defined nutritional pathways where it is clear how to add natural supplements to bypass imbalances. My personal opinion is that running tests that result in a laundry list of mutations without a way to use nutritional support to bypass these mutations is not ethical. I feel that whether you have a test that gives you 30 or 1000 or 5000 markers this is still only a fraction of the total number of genes in your body and frankly having more markers is not the issue. The real question is whether the information that you have is in a pathway that has been characterized so you know what to do to help restore your body to health.

Again, to reiterate, changes in the DNA that can impair its function are called SNPs. This stands for single nucleotide polymorphisms. SNPs are single changes that can occur in any portion of the DNA that modify the ability of the DNA to function. You can think of a SNP as a slight imperfection in your car that can affect its performance. If your car that you have been given, the car that needs to last your entire lifetime has a weak clamp holding your tailpipe in place that could be considered a SNP. You may have a weak clamp in your car, as compared to another individual who received a car without a weak clamp. That other individual does not have a SNP in a location where you unfortunately do. A weak tailpipe clamp might be considered a less severe SNP or mutation. On the other hand a defect that causes your engine to spontaneously catch on fire would be a significant SNP or mutation. There are times where what may seem insignificant, actually has the potential to become a more serious matter. Recently over a million high end vehicles were recalled for a missing battery cable cover. While at first glance this seems minor, the lack of the battery cover potentially caused cars to catch on fire. Bottom line, we are not just concerned about the number of SNP or mutations that your car has, but also the type of SNP and the effect that mutation has on the safety and ability to drive that car. This again highlights why I feel so strongly about only looking for SNPs where you understand their impact, where you know what pathway they are located, and where you know how to bypass and remedy the situation. Finally, and I will talk about this more later, it is not just the car you are given for life, but also the way you drive it that affects its survival. You may be given the most high end vehicle, with no defects or mutations at all, but if you drive it at excessive speeds and never service the vehicle and are reckless the result will be a serious or fatal accident despite the quality of the car.

The nutritional pathway that this program focuses on, is something I call "The Methylation Cycle". The methylation cycle is a well-defined nutritional pathway in the body such that it is very clear where support can be used to bypass mutations.

Since it is a key concept, I reiterate that the field of nutrigenomics is the study of how natural products and supplements can interact with particular genes to decrease the risk of disease. By looking at changes in the DNA in these nutritional pathways it enables us to make supplement choices based on your particular genetics, rather than using the same support for every individual regardless of their unique needs. Knowledge of imbalances in nutritional genetic pathways allows you to utilize combinations of nutrients, foods and natural nucleotides to bypass mutations and restore proper pathway function. However, before we get to supplement suggestions to help you on your road to health and wellness, it is important to understand that most mutations or SNP variations that are revealed are NOT "all or none mutations". In other words, if you or your loved one has a mutation or SNP variation, it does not mean that the activity of the gene is completely "off". It may simply mean it functions at a lower efficiency. When you look at the suggested nutritional support, you are working to increase the ability of the entire Methylation Cycle to run properly, keeping in mind that it has been functioning to some degree in spite of any mutations in particular genes.

Just as the physical location of your hometown will not change, your genetics will not change over time either. For this reason nutrigenomic test results will serve as a Roadmap for your future.

Knowledge of your genetics is like having an ultrasound that allows you to see inside your own individual DNA. This is important information that can be used to help avoid potential health issues. Suggestions that are made may be valid today, as well as next week, next year or ten years from now. Once you slowly implement a supplementation regimen that is designed to bybass the mutations, this helps in supporting the Methylation Cycle to function properly.

Nutrigenomic test results that look at SNPs in your DNA should help to put your mind at ease by giving you suggestions that you can act on. Nutrigenomics is a form of genetic testing that supplies information that can translate into positive constructive action. I see the ultimate goal of nutrigenomic testing to serve as a guide toward proper supplementation to bypass genetic weaknesses identified by SNP results.

Another way to look at SNPs in less technical terms is to go back to the concept of thinking of SNPs as defects in your car. At any time these defects can create havoc such that your car gets stuck on the road, blows out a tire or creates an accident on a highway. If you start to think about the biochemical pathways in your body as roads and traffic circles you can see how your car being stuck in the middle of a lane prevents the flow of traffic on that particular roadway.

I see and define The Methylation Cycle is a series of four connected traffic circles. Your body needs to navigate these four traffic circles in order to process nutrients properly. As an example, if these traffic circles are not functioning as intended non ideal compounds can build up in your system such as high homocysteine. High levels of homocysteine have been linked to atherosclerosis (hardening of the arteries), heart attaches, stroke, blood clots and possibly Alzheimer's disease.

The goal is to compensate for the defects in your car, in other words to bypass the SNPs in your body, so that the four traffic circles that are part of the Methylation Cycle flow properly such that there are no blocks on these roadways. This helps to support the body so that nonideal compounds do not build up; additionally that the desired products of these pathways are produced.

With the knowledge of where your nutrigenomic weaknesses are, we can predict the places accidents are likely to be located in your traffic circles. It is then possible to use appropriate nutritional support to bypass the accidents, to take alternate routes around the trouble spots so that the products of these four traffic circles are what you desire and nonideal compounds are avoided.

By using nutrigenomic testing that focuses precisely on the Methylation Cycle, it is possible to determine the SNPs in this particular pathway. While this does not give us the information about the remainder of the 25,000 genes, what it does is to let us know what is going on with a well characterized set of traffic circles where we know the end products that are desired and where we know how to use supplements to bypass issues. We know the actual locations we are interested in. We know the exact intersection/cross streets where we want to know if there is a traffic issue or not. So ahead of time we have 'eyes on the ground' placed at those precise intersections looking to see if there is an issue or not along those highways, necessitating that you take a detour to get around the traffic accident. SNP information allows you to discern between a minor fender bender, a serious fatal accident or a car stopped by the side of the road to ask for directions or one whose radiator has overheated.

There are several reasons why this program focuses on the Methylation Cycle. First, as you will read about in the next section the Methylation Cycle has a critical editing function in the body that has the capacity to get around other SNPs in different regions of your DNA. As I will discuss in a few moments, the Methylation Cycle helps to serve as the built in mechanic for the car you have been given in this life. Even if your car has more defects that someone else's, with proper functioning of the Methylation Cycle you can compensate for the state of the car you were given. Second, the Methylation Cycle is a combination of four well defined nutritional pathways. As I already stated, I do not believe in genetic testing if you have no positive course of action to deploy once you obtain the results. Aside from the critical role that the Methylation Cycle plays as your body's personal mechanic, the compounds in these cycles are well known, understood and nutritional support to bypass imbalances in these cycles are well known. So you have a concrete path to follow to get around issues in the Methylation Cycle.

Finally, I feel that it makes logical sense to comprehensively look at one region. If you wanted to travel from your hometown to my rural town in Maine you would need a map with detailed directions. This would be especially important if certain roads along the way were closed due to construction, bridges out because of flooding, or road detours. It would help to have a detailed map drawn for you that took all of these specific situations into account. Your nutrigenomic test tells you where the "construction" sites are located, which bridges are out and where detours are on your individualized map. With this knowledge you can put together an analysis that will help you to get from your hometown to my hometown in Maine without getting stuck in a ditch or lost on a detour. The more information you have about specific genes in this particular pathway the easier it is to construct your personal map. This is analogous to having the model of your car, knowing how many miles per gallon you get, how often you feel you need to stop at a rest area and when you need to fill your tank or take a break from driving. With this information you are in a better position to plan your trip. This is different from other tests that may tell you where your hometown is located and your destination lies on a map, but without any of the specific information between those two points. Without the details, you do not know if the route you may choose has been closed, if the bridge is out, of if there is a detour that will add more time to your travel. Given only a starting and stopping point, on the map means the rest of the trip may simply be guesswork. Focusing on the Methylation Cycle allows you to look comprehensively at a very critical pathway in the body and from that construct a personal Roadmap to Health and wellness.

Nutrigenomics is just one aspect of the factors that determine your health. As I talked about earlier, it is not just the car you are given (the genetics you are born with) it is also how you drive that car that plays a role in your health. How you care for that car, how often you service it, how fast you drive it all impact how long that car will last and how well it will function. I see complex health conditions as multifactorial in nature. That means that while your nutrigenomics are a piece of the puzzle they are not the whole picture. The environmental burden of toxins you are exposed to, along with infectious agents (viruses, bacteria, fungal infections, yeast) and the stress on your system all impact your overall health.

I believe that most health conditions in society today are multifactorial conditions, meaning that a number of circumstances need to go awry simultaneously for nonideal health to manifest. Multifactorial conditions stem from underlying genetic susceptibility combined with assaults from environmental stressors and infectious agents. Basic parameters like age and gender, along with other genetic and environmental factors play a role in the onset of non-ideal health. Infections combined with excessive environmental burdens will generally only lead to serious problems with health if they occur in individuals with the appropriate genetic susceptibility.

Personalized nutrigenomic screening is one clear, definitive way to evaluate the genetic contribution of multifactorial conditions. **Part of what makes the Methylation Cycle so unique and so critical for our health is that mutations in this**

pathway have the capability to impair all of these factors. This would suggest that if an individual has enough mutations or weaknesses in this pathway, it may be sufficient to cause multifactorial health issues. Methylation Cycle mutations can lead to chronic infectious diseases, increased environmental toxin burdens and have secondary effects on the expression of other genes.

Speeding Through Life: the Gas Pedal is Stuck

One of the key starting points for this program, in parallel with the focus on the Methylation Cycle is the recognition of the role of glutamate and GABA (gamma-aminobutyric acid) in chronic neurological conditions. In many cases, especially when my focus was adults in my private practice, merely working to balance glutamate and GABA was sufficient for a return to health. Excess glutamate has been illustrated to be a factor in a number of neurological conditions including Parkinson's disease, Multiple Sclerosis, Huntington's disease, ALS (Lou Gehrig's disease), fibromyalgia and chronic fatigue syndrome amongst others. Balancing glutamate and GABA is the first step of the program for autism and there too, **a number of individuals find that glutamate/GABA balance is all that is needed to relieve a number of symptoms.**

To understand this concept it is important to realize that excess glutamate relative to GABA can over excite your nerves.

Glutamate works with calcium to stimulate your nervous system. Some stimulation is a good thing, but too much stimulation can leave you feeling nervous, twitchy and unable to sleep. The goal is to keep glutamate in balance so that you gain the benefits from it without having so much that your system is unbalanced.

One way to visualize the impact of excess glutamate in the body is like a car whose gas pedal is stuck, pressed to the floor. Speeding through life, without the ability to put on the brakes virtually ensures that you will either experience a major crash due to excessive speed or eventually run out of gas. Think of glutamate as the gas and GABA as the brake pedal. While you need the gas pedal to move forward in life, you also require the ability to use the brake as needed to be certain that you're able to moderate your speed.

Recognize that we do need glutamate, it helps us to think and process information. But too much glutamate will exhaust your nerves to the point of creating health issues. Glutamate is considered an "excitotoxin". Excitotoxins are compounds that have the ability to overexcite nerves to death. Before you even start to work on your Methylation Cycle you can begin by working on your glutamate/GABA balance. Look to eliminate food and supplement sources from your diet that serve to increase glutamate beyond a healthy level. Look to support with nutrients that help to calm the nervous system including GABA, valerian root, theanine, pycnogenol, grape seed extract, resveratrol and CoQ10.

As with glutamate, calcium is something your system needs. But too much calcium will work with glutamate to overexcite your nervous system. One way to look at the interaction between calcium and glutamate is that glutamate is the gun and calcium is the bullet. In experiments looking at the impact of minerals on excitotoxin death it was found that *"Calcium, it appeared, was the culprit. Apparently glutamate opened a special channel designed to allow calcium to enter the neuron, and it was calcium that triggered the cell to die...It appeared that excitotoxins, including glutamate and aspartate work by opening calcium channels, at least on certain subtypes of receptors. When those neurotransmitters are allowed to come into contact with the receptor in too high a concentration or for too long a period of time, the calcium channel gets stuck in the open position allowing calcium to pour into the cell in large amounts"* (Russell Blaylock, Excitotoxins the Taste that Kills). Thus, you want to strike a healthy balance in terms of the level of calcium support you are using. Look to support with magnesium, zinc and lithium which may help to balance excess calcium in the system.

According to Dr.Russell Blaylock, we are often unaware of the issues of excess glutamate until more than 80% of our neurons have been impaired. *"What is so unusual about these diseases is* *that most of the people who are affected by them have lived perfectly healthy lives up until the time the disease strikes, which is usually later in life.. ..The puzzle of what causes these particular neurons to start dying after decades of normal function has intrigued neuroscientists for many years...evidence began to appear indicating that even though the symptoms do not appear until the later years the pathological destruction of neurons begins much earlier, even decades earlier...the symptoms of Parkinson's disease do not manifest themselves until over 80 to 90% of the neurons in the involved nuclei have died. The neurons didn't all suddenly die at the same time, rather they slowly and silently deteriorated over many years. The same is true for Alzheimer's disease. **This is why prevention is so important.**"*

Addressing imbalances in the glutamate/GABA ratio as well as the calcium to magnesium ratio is what I consider the starting point, or Step One of this program. Even in the absence of nutrigenomic SNP information you can begin to work on addressing excitotoxicity in your system. This is a critical ongoing way of life, to keep glutamate and calcium in balance as you move forward to work on the other aspects of multiifactorial health conditions.

CHAPTER 8

The Perfect Storm: Multifactorial Conditions

The role of glutamate in overexciting nerves is just one piece of the puzzle in terms of the multiple factors that impact health. Sometimes, a number of seemingly unrelated events occur simultaneously, resulting in disaster. A prime example of this was the death of Princess Diana...if she had been wearing her seatbelt, if the car hadn't been speeding, if the driver hadn't presumably been drinking, if the paparazzi weren't chasing the car, if they hadn't driven into a narrow tunnel . . . if there had been a way to eliminate any one of those factors, that tragedy might have been averted. The multitude of factors that must occur to create complex health conditions can be viewed in a similar fashion. Without a particular combination of genetic mutations, heavy metal toxicities, chronic viral infection, underlying bacterial infections, and excitotoxin damage leading to a negative cascade of neurological events, we have better overall health.

In my experience, achieving optimal health requires recognition of all of the factors that can create a perfect storm. We've been taught that health management is just a matter of taking one pill, but it's far more complex than that. I want you to begin to see health conditions differently so that you can individualize the approach and access what you need to do for optimal health. In this protocol, I take into account a range of factors contributing to all health conditions, including genetic, environmental, and toxic burden. The protocol aims to suggest the key nutrients needed to address these conditions and manage the factors undermining health.

- **Excitotoxins:** These are chemicals present in many common foods that overstimulate brain chemistry via the neurotransmitters and nerve receptors. This over-stimulation can trigger nerve cell death, which results in poor signaling, and nerve damage. Excitoxins include ingredients such as monosodium glutamate, aspartame, glutamate, hydrolyzed protein, and aspartic acid.

- **Heavy metal toxicity:** Arising from environmental exposures and compounded by metals in vaccines, heavy metals disrupt the immune system and the digestive organs, reduce energy, impair cognitive and neurological function and weaken the individual.

- **Chronic viral and bacterial infections:** Arising from environmental exposures, these chronic infections disrupt the immune, digestive, and respiratory systems, thus undermining the body's ability to maintain and repair itself.

- **Methylation deficiencies:** Imbalances in the Methylation Cycle which is a key cellular pathway that promotes detoxification, controls inflammation, and balances the neurotransmitters, can result in mood and emotional shifts as well as liver, pancreas, stomach, intestinal, adrenal, thyroid, and hormonal imbalances.

Predisposing genetics, exposure to environmental toxins, the infectious disease burden and stress all contribute to our propensity for non ideal health. Knowledge of where the mutations are in the Methylation Cycle and supporting to bypass those SNPs is one piece of a larger health program. Working to balance glutamate and GABA is yet another factor. Working to address environmental toxins as well as better microbial balance in the gut are additional positive steps that can be taken on the Roadmap to Health.

Overall, my husband and I have been very fortunate with the health of our three daughters. This is in spite of some very non ideal genetics and some unfortunate situations. The fact that all three daughters are all doing quite well helps to exemplify that a number of factors need to go awry simultaneously to create that perfect storm of health problems. Multifactorial conditions require underlying genetic susceptibility along with exposure to environmental toxins, stress and infectious agents in the absence of supplementation to support positive epigenetic influences. The genetics from my husband's side of the family are not stellar. His paternal grandmother had Alzheimer's his maternal grandfather died of ALS, his father had a heart attack at an early age and his mother had several brain tumors. In terms of his parents, a testament to a healthy lifestyle is that both survived those major medical events and are healthy and vibrant to this day. Needless to say some of the genes that my girls inherited are not pristine. In addition, one of them is a sulfite sensitive asthmatic and until we were aware of that condition 911 was called more than once for respiratory issues. One of the other daughters had a severe case of mononucleosis and streptococcus such that her tonsils were so enlarged her throat was almost entirely closed off. And the third daughter had such a severe concussion that she was unable to read or drive for months. Yet, in spite of less than ideal genetics, and these additional health incidents all are healthy, bright and successful. Why are they not riddled with chronic health issues, with CFS, with ADD or glutamate related problems? I believe the answer is living in a clean less toxic environment combined with the use of nutritional supplements to bypass mutations from a very young age.

Before any of our girls were old enough to swallow pills we would crush the supplements on a spoon and add honey and have them lick the nutrients off the spoon. I expect they thought that everyone was raised to take multiple supplements daily. My youngest recently started her own vitamin company directed towards the needs of dancers, once she realized that not everyone had grown up taking supplements to support their body. Nutritional supplementation can have a major positive impact on your health, especially if you haven't been given the best car on the lot for your vehicle to drive for life.

We want to be paying attention, not only to the SNPs and ways to bypass those SNPs, but also to our exposure to environmental toxins and how we support our systems to deal with infectious agents so that we can overcome all of these factors for better health.

CHAPTER 9

Navigating the Traffic Circles

What I call the "Methylation Cycle" is actually the intersection of four traffic circles. Traffic circles can be difficult to navigate. If you don't already know where you are supposed to be exiting you can find yourself in the absolute wrong lane and need to traverse the circle more than once to actually get off at the desired location. The Methylation Cycle is more complex in that all four traffic circles are connected to each other and each one produces critical components that are needed by your body. The combination of two of these circles is well known; the addition of the other two circles is part of what influences the supplement choices for this program. Combining all four of these circles into the Methylation Cycle has allowed me to think about these pathways in a unique manner and define supplementation in a different way. Part of the success of this program is recognizing that what you do in one traffic circle can influence the others.

I will not get too technical in this book. There are a large number of resources I have generated (books, workbook, DVD, PPTs, articles) that go into detail once you are ready to learn more. Getting your arms around this program is like driving a car. My goal in this book is simply for you to understand that this is a car you really need to learn how to drive, in order to have a better Roadmap to health for you and your entire family. In describing these traffic circles I will give you the bare minimum scientific information you need to understand how critical it is for your body to be able to navigate the Methylation Cycle.

- The first traffic circle involves one of the many building blocks for proteins, an amino acid called methionine. This first circle is aptly named the methionine cycle. This cycle helps to convert homocysteine back to methionine. Buildup of homocysteine has been linked to stroke, heart disease and Alzheimer's disease among other health conditions. The ability to convert homocysteine to methionine is clearly important for health. If you consider that heart disease, Alzheimer's, and stroke are all leading causes of death, it is obvious that this is a traffic circle you don't want to ignore. Not only do you want to decrease homocysteine levels, generating methionine is something your system needs. Lack of methionine has been linked to fatty liver disease and depression and has been used to help offset toxicity due to certain chemical poisoning, for asthma and allergies as well as playing a role in decreasing gray hair.

- The second circle that is well known to be tied to the methionine cycle is the folate cycle. Folate is simply a B vitamin. So, just as methionine is a building block of proteins that you eat every day, folate is a B vitamin that is found in green leafy vegetables. The folate cycle is linked to the methionine cycle so that they can be envisioned as two gears. The gears are linked and help to drive each other around the circle. The functioning of the folate/methionine cycles drives the regeneration of methionine from homocysteine through the use and conversion of B vitamins.

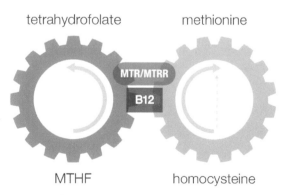

When there are certain mutations in the Methylation Cycle the folate portion cannot function optimally. Since these two cycles are matched together like gears that drive each other's movement, you can see how Methylation Cycle

SNPs can have a direct negative impact on the balance of homocysteine and methionine. In addition, imbalances in this folate/methionine cycle have been linked to everything from neural tube defects, miscarriages, cleft palate, anemia to cancer.

The central point where the first two cycles meet is a step that requires vitamin B12. The need to support B12 is a critical aspect of this program. I will talk more about B12 and the special types of B12 you can consider as well as the importance of lithium with respect to B12 levels. However for the moment, all I ask is that you keep the need for B12 in mind and how it sits at the juncture of the first two cycles.

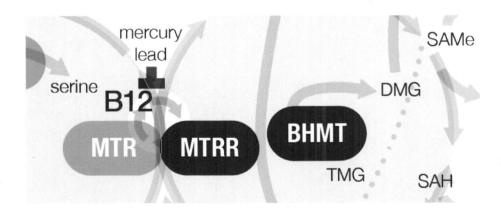

- The third traffic circle that is part of the Methylation Cycle is the BH4 cycle. BH4 stands for tetrahydrobiopterin. I do not expect you to even try to pronounce that. But I do want you to understand why BH4 is so important. BH4 is what your body uses to help make the 'feel good' compounds in your body, serotonin and dopamine. Most antidepressants on the market today rely on the need for serotonin and dopamine but do not consider the role of BH4. Your body converts tryptophan (from turkey) to serotonin with the help of BH4. Serotonin makes you feel content and satisfied, like a purring cat. Lack of serotonin has been tied to depression. BH4 also helps you make dopamine from another amino acid, tyrosine. Dopamine is the compound that gives you that sense of satisfaction from achievement that gives you motivation and prevents you from being a couch potato. Lack of dopamine is associated with Parkinson's disease and other movement disorders and imbalances in dopamine have been linked to ADD/ADHD. Together with serotonin, having healthy dopamine levels is a key to feeling happy, content, satisfied, focused and motivated.

Certain mutations in the Methylation Cycle may impair the ability to generate healthy BH4 levels. This fact ties together the BH4 traffic circle to the first two traffic circles we already spoke about (methionine and folate). BH4 levels are further compromised by environmental toxins including aluminum, lead and mercury. So, underlying SNPs in the Methylation Cycle combined with toxic chemicals can further diminish much needed BH4 levels. In addition, bacterial infections in the body can throw off the balance of BH4. So adding in infectious agents along with toxins and SNPs helps to create the ingredients for that perfect storm of BH4 deficiency. Low levels of BH4 can then cause a range of problems including feeling depressed, unmotivated, a lack of focus and movement issues.

• The final traffic circle that is a part of the Methylation Cycle is the urea cycle. This is the cycle that helps the body get rid of ammonia, which is toxic, and convert it to urea which can be excreted. Lack of BH4 not only impacts dopamine and serotonin as discussed above, but also plays a role in the urea cycle. BH4 helps to generate products that cause less oxidative damage. In the absence of sufficient BH4 more oxygen related damaging compounds are produced from the urea cycle that can cause neurological inflammation.

By this point you should be able to see that the Methylation Cycle is a central pathway in the body that is particularly amenable to nutrigenomic screening for genetic weaknesses. The result of decreased activity in this pathway causes a shortage of critical functional groups in the body called methyl groups that serve a variety of important functions. **In general, single mutations**

or biomarkers are generally perceived as indicators for specific health issues. However, it is possible that for a number of health conditions, it may be necessary to look at the *entire* Methylation Cycle as a biomarker for underlying genetic susceptibility for nonideal health. It may require expanding the view of a biomarker beyond the restriction of a mutation in a single gene to a mutation somewhere in an entire pathway of interconnected function.

Four Components of the Methylation Cycle

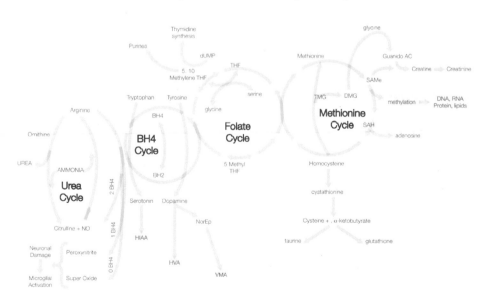

CHAPTER 10

Your Body's Mechanic

The concept of "one mutation, one disease" originated in 1948, when the Nobel Prize laureate, Dr. Linus Pauling, began a new age in biomedical science with his historic work on sickle cell anemia. Pauling was the first person to characterize a disease at a molecular level illustrating that a mutation in a particular gene could cause an identifiable disease. A cause and effect; he had identified the "diseased gene" responsible for sickle cell anemia. The finding of a single gene for an individual disease sparked the hope and imagination of scientists and researchers. The knowledge of the gene involved could be used to diagnose and treat disease; the implication was that disease-causing genes could be found for every imaginable condition. And so began the equivalent of the "California gold rush" in pursuit of human genes. This would lay the groundwork for the Human Genome Project (the defining of the complete human genetic code) and today's DNA based genetic tests. What was not understood at the time was the "one gene one disease" relationship is only applicable in certain instances. Many genes have multiple functions and other environmental and infectious components that can impact upon the ability of a genetic defect to ultimately manifest as disease. Yet at the time it seemed as if we had the explanation not only for infectious diseases but also for genetic diseases. Armed with this knowledge it would pave the way for therapeutic treatments for even inherited disorders.

How naïve we were. The fact that in 1953, the actual structure of DNA, as the material comprising our genomes, was **first** elucidated should have been an inkling that we were at the beginning of a long journey rather than at its end. It was not until 1968 that the notion of RNA as an "information molecule" was first proposed. Different types of RNA in the cell were first identified thirty years ago and concepts for manipulating RNA to influence gene expression have only emerged since the 1980's. We are living in an exciting time from the standpoint of medical breakthroughs. Just as the computer has evolved from a 943 cubic foot giant to a laptop unit that can be carried in a backpack, so too the fields of molecular medicine and nutrigenomics have first begun to evolve.

In single gene disorders a mutation or defect exists in one gene, which results in the faulty production of its protein product. This would be analogous to having a defective concrete mixture that was used to pour the foundation for your new home. Every bag of concrete mix that was received from the cement factory contains this "mutation" such that it would be impossible for us to find a *single* bag that does not contain our "concrete mutation". The end result of this faulty concrete mixture would be a foundation with holes or cracks or air pockets, your home's version of a "faulty protein product" based on a defective gene, the "concrete mix gene". This one defective component thus affects the stability of the entire new home, which is to be built upon the unstable foundation.

A classic example of what has been perceived to be a single gene disorder is the case of cystic fibrosis. If an individual carries particular CFTR gene SNPs they are likely to have the disease. The following quote illustrates that things are not always as simple as they might seem in terms of treatment, even when the genetic defect is well characterized. *"Back in 1989, a giddy optimism swept over researchers, patients, and the public when the cystic fibrosis (CF) genome and its abnormality - a single error in a quarter of a million genetic letters - became one of the first discovered. The NIH made CF a priority, and researchers at various institutions and pharmaceutical companies moved quickly on the news. One year later, two excited research teams corrected CF cells in the lab by adding normal copies of the gene, and high expectations reigned for a drug that would replace the defective gene. However, the CF protein turned out to be too complex, unwieldy, and toxic to be made into a drug. Moreover, vectors that triggered the body's natural immune system slowed any progress in a gene therapy approach. Fourteen years later, the hoped–for genetics cure is still considered close to 10 years away"* (Richards, L., Modern Drug Discovery, June, 2004).

This was written a decade ago, and we are still far from a definitive molecular treatment for cystic fibrosis. Yet from this quote we can begin to see the logic and thinking behind the molecular medicine approach to disease. Methods used by standard medicine to isolate appropriate drugs may not be well suited to address the multifactorial nature of many of these diseases. *"…the most significant problem in relation to target* (drug) *discovery is the multifactorial nature of the chronic diseases that are presently the focus of many pharmaceutical and biotechnology companies"* (Lindsay, Nature Reviews Drug Discovery).

In comparison, recent findings in the field of nutrition suggest that answers to some of these complex diseases may lie in the use of natural supplements. Supplements may be helpful for genetically well-defined conditions even if we do not understand the precise mode of action of these nutritional supplements.

The use of the nutritional supplement glutathione has shown initial promise in helping to curb the severity of cystic fibrosis (Richards, L., Modern Drug Discovery). Preliminary trials using glutathione in cystic fibrosis patients demonstrated that the glutathione was able to significantly lower the level of oxidative stress in these individuals (Roum,J., Journal of Applied Physiology).   As Valerie Hudson states with respect to glutathione, *__Though not a "cure"__ for CF (as the underlying genetic defect remains), and though not a "panacea" for all CF-related ills (for some of those ills are not caused by GSH deficiency), it is nevertheless a therapeutic approach that calls for serious clinical investigation"* (Hudson, V., Free Radical Biology and Medicine).

Recently, a second supplement, the herb curcumin has emerged as a potential tool to help offset some of the symptoms of this genetic disorder. In animal models curcumin supplementation was able to have a positive impact on symptoms of cystic fibrosis (Egan,Science). In this study the curcumin treated mice regained nearly normal nasal function. Additional research in the past year has shown that utilizing curcumin packaged in a special manner enhances delivery and expands the applicability of this approach (Cartiera, Mol Pharm).

So in spite of the genetic defect, we are able to add a component that alters the expression or manifestation of the mutation. If we go back to our "defective concrete gene" example this would be equivalent to adding a hardening agent to the defective cement mixture that allows us to overcome the mutation and have a more solid foundation.

This points to what many scientists have observed, that having a particular gene is not a guarantee that you will express the associated trait regardless of the "one gene/ specific disease" scenario. The ability to turn on or off genes also plays an important role in what we observe. This is what is known as epigenetics. *"Epigenetics is to genetics as the dark matter in the universe is to the stars; we know it's important, but it's difficult to see...What we're thinking now is that, in addition to genetic variation, there may be epigenetic variation that is very important in human disease"* (Andrew Feinberg, Johns Hopkins School of Medicine).

You have about 25,000 genes all of which may have SNPs or mutations that impact their function. The body is a beautiful organism and has a system in place to help correct or compensate for mutations in our DNA. This system uses methylation to turn on and turn off genes by a mechanism called epigenetics. **The reason I focus on the Methylation Cycle and the reason that the nutrigenomic test I use looks solely at genes in this pathway is that mutations in these genes not only affect the function of the genes carrying those mutations, they also affect the global editing function that the body relies on to help to compensate for issues in the remainder of the 25,000 genes.** Having the Methylation Cycle function optimally and bypassing SNPs in this pathway allows the global editing function in your body to help to correct issues with **any number of other genes** in the system. THIS is why this pathway is so critical for health and wellness.

"With the completion of the Human Genome Project, we have a nearly complete list of the genes needed to produce a human. However, the situation is far more complex than a simple catalogue of genes. Of equal importance is a second system that cells use to determine when and where a particular gene will be expressed during development. This system (DNA methylation) *is overlaid on DNA in the form of epigenetic marks that are heritable during cell division but do not alter the DNA....**The importance of DNA methylation is emphasized by the growing number of human diseases that are known to occur when this epigenetic information is not properly established and/or maintained**...*"(Keith Robertson, Nature Review Genetics).

The Methylation Cycle is the system the body uses to edit and correct problems with other genes. Regardless of how many other SNPs there are in the 25,000 or so other genes in the body, since those genes are regulated by methylation, then having your Methylation Cycle in balance gives you the tools you need to help to turn on or off those other genes.

This process is called epigenetics. While your DNA will not change over your lifetime, your epigenetics can change. The prefix "epi" literally means "over or attached to". When it comes to **epi**genetics this means attaching a group to your DNA. Again, your DNA will not change, but the groups that can be attached to your DNA *can* change, and more importantly can influence the function of your DNA. Epigenetics serve as an editing function that helps to turn on and off your other genes. Epigenetics gives your body a way to compensate for problems in the DNA that you have inherited. Epigenetics is literally defined as "heritable changes in gene expression patterns that occur without changes in DNA sequence".

In my opinion, the reason the pathway that we focus on, the 'Methylation Cycle' is so critical to health and well-being is that SNPs or mutations in *this* portion of your DNA affect your editing function as well as that portion of the DNA itself. This is such an important concept that I want you to be sure you really understand the magnitude of this situation.

While the term may seem intimidating, a methyl group is actually just a group of small molecules, similar in size to a water molecule (H_2O). Water is a key to life as are methyl groups critical for health and well-being. Methyl groups are simply "CH_3" groups; they contain 'H' like in water and a 'C' like in coal or diamonds. However, these very basic molecules serve integral functions; they are moved around in the body to turn on or off genes.

One way to look at the role of methyl groups is that they serve as your own personal mechanic for your body, helping to repair and direct functions in your body. If we think about your body like a car then let's assume that you have just one car that you need to maintain over the course of your life, with the help of your own personal mechanic. The longer you have that car the more outdated it will become. Over the course of a lifetime the car body will accumulate rust and can rot out. Tires may wear out and the engine may need an overhaul.

Alternatively the problems may be less complicated such as the need for more wiper fluid or simply to keep the car filled with gas and to regularly change the oil. In any case your personal mechanic ensures that your car keeps running, that it can stay on the road...in this case on the road to health. However, if your mechanic is unable to function, then all of these issues will start to accumulate over the course of the lifetime of your car. The rust may get so bad that car components fall off like your muffler or the tires become so worn that it is impossible to navigate a turn without the fear of blowing a tire. In the absence of your mechanic you have no way to repair all of the large and small problems that arise with your car to the point where your car can no longer function.

I truly want to be certain that you understand this critical concept of the global editing function of the Methylation Cycle. Another analogy that helps to illustrate the crucial role of this pathway is to view the function of methyl groups as analogous to the editing function on your computer. If we think about your body like a computer then you have just one computer that you need to maintain over the course of your life. The longer you have that computer the more outdated it will become. Over the course of a lifetime many of the keys may become stuck or broken. You may drop the computer and damage its function or spill your coffee on it. However, the editing function of the computer remains intact and compensates for these broken keys, misspelled words, and sticky space bars due to accidents of wear and tear. In the absence of this editing function, assume that these 'misspells' are accumulated in your body over the course of your life. If the editing function is impaired then you have no way to get around these misspelled words and other issues that affect your ability to function. Over your lifetime you will accumulate so many misspelled words, missed keys, etc. that at a certain point it would be impossible to read a 'document' amidst all of these mistakes.

You can start to see why the proper functioning of the pathway that serves to direct your genes is so important. In addition to the editing of genes, this pathway also serves more direct roles in your body and is thus critical for overall health. While there are several particular sites in this pathway where blocks can occur as a result of genetic weaknesses, thankfully supplementation with appropriate foods and nutrients can help to bypass these mutations to allow for restored function of this pathway.

By testing to look at mutations in the DNA for this Methylation Cycle it is possible to draw a personalized map for each individual's imbalances which may impact upon their health. Once the precise areas of genetic fragility have been identified, it is then possible to target appropriate nutritional supplementation of these pathways to optimize the functioning of these crucial biochemical processes. There are specific places in the cycle where support can be added. This support helps to bypass mutations in the pathway in a similar manner to the way you might take a detour on a highway. We can look at mutations in this pathway as analogous to a collision that has totally shut down traffic going in one direction on a highway. Support to bypass mutations in this pathway is like taking an alternate route to avoid the accident on the highway. Thus, the use of key nutrients or foods can aid in helping to bypass methylation cycle mutations and help restore function to this pathway

It does not mean that every individual with mutations in this pathway will have one or more nonideal health condition. It may be a necessary but not a sufficient condition. Most health conditions in society today are multifactorial in nature. There are genetic components, infectious components and environmental components. A certain threshold or body burden needs to be met for each of these factors in order for multifactorial disease to occur.

A key component to charting your personal Roadmap to health is understanding the importance of the Methylation Cycle for overall health and wellness. Understanding that mutations in the group of genes involved in this cycle can not only impair a specific gene's function but also have the ability to impair our global editing system. **The Methylation Cycle is our fall back system that helps to compensate for mutations in our DNA in general.**

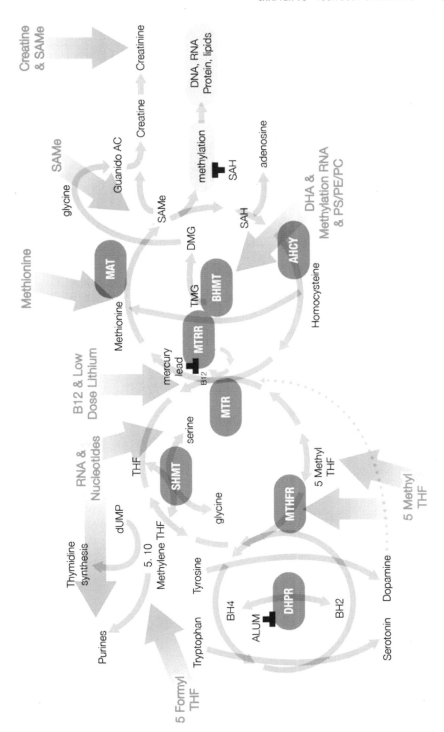

CHAPTER 11

Inheritance and Ancestry

Just as you have one car, one set of DNA genetics that you inherit to last you an entire lifetime, you also inherit the epigenetic changes to your DNA. The extent to which your mother or father, or grandparent's DNA were methylated is passed down from generation to generation. You in turn will pass down the extent of epigenetic methylation that your DNA contains. While you cannot change your DNA, you can change your epigenetics. I am always reminded of the line in the movie *A Knights Tale* when I think about epigenetics. When John Thatcher tells William that yes, you can change your stars. Your DNA is the lot in life you were cast genetically, but epigenetics allow you to change your stars. Equally important, IF you change your stars, and bypass mutations so that your epigenetics function properly, then this change will be passed on to future generations.

This is an important concept and helps to highlight why the Methylation Cycle is so important to health and well-being and plays a role in so many health conditions. The DNA that is part of your editing system (your epigenetic system) is part of a well known nutritional pathway. This is wonderful on the part of Mother Nature, that a system that is so critical for health is amenable to bypassing mutations through natural supplements and is a well defined system so we know where the accidents are on this highway to health and how to detour around them. This epigenetic system puts methyl groups on our DNA. While the DNA itself cannot change over our lifetimes, the positioning of the methyl groups on the DNA can, and those groups help to affect the activity of that DNA. The placement of these methyl groups on the DNA is something that is passed down from generation to generation. If you change your own stars, if you start to bypass mutations in your Methylation Cycle then you make a positive difference for the next generation. Unlike your DNA which you inherit and you cannot change, you have a second chance when it comes to epigenetics. Many families have a history of autism, bipolar disorder, stroke, Parkinson's. The mutations in the DNA that may predispose you to these conditions are inherited as are the methyl groups attached to the DNA that alter its function. By supporting healthy Methylation Cycle function in your body you open the door to changing the methyl groups that are attached to the DNA, changing the inheritance pattern of epigenetics and changing your stars and that of your future generations.

The genetics that predispose to imbalances in the Methylation Cycle come from both parents. And the epigenetic changes to that DNA are also inherited from the father, the mother as well as grandparents. There are approximately 25,000 genes in your body. DNA has two strands, like a ladder with two long supporting pieces that are held together by the rungs. One of those support structures comes from each parent, so it is easy to see how both the mother and the father contribute equally to the DNA of the child. And why, if for instance your child has autism or ADD that I am suggesting that both parents may also have predisposing imbalances in *their* SNPs for their own Methylation Cycle.

Simply by the small modifications made to these 25,000 genes, these epigenetic tags increase the patterns of DNA to 50 to 100 times its actual size.

Epigenetics helps to explain how identical twins, with the same DNA can have very different health conditions that are related to the extent of their methylation. The appearance of Systemic Lupus Erythematosus (lupus) in one of two identical twins, has been tied to differences between the two in terms of their DNA methylation.

It is well known that diet and nutrition can affect epigenetics and health. A classic experiment to demonstrate this fact used genetically identical sets of mice that were given specific nutrients during pregnancy. The mice who received nutrients that are part of the Methylation Cycle had pups with normal weight and healthy brown fur. The genetically identical mice who lacked methylation support had pups that were obese, had greater health issues and lighter fur. Using genetically identical animal models it is clear that diet and nutrition are able to influence epigenetics.

Since epigenetic changes to the DNA are influenced by nutrition it might be a little more difficult to envision how the epigenetic influence can come from both parents. Unlike the inheritance of DNA and SNPs where each parent contributes one of the supporting structures of the DNA ladder It would seem logical that only the mother who carries the growing child, would play a solitary role with respect to the epigenetic aspect.

However, when it comes to epigenetics it is not just about the mom! Recent studies have demonstrated that epigenetic changes in sperm are carried forward transgenerationally. Thus it is not just the mom, or the dad but even the grandfather that can influence the pattern of epigenetics. This research found that both the eggs and sperm from *even* great grandparents could be passed on to their children and grandchildren by a process called transgenerational epigenetic inheritance. So that the way in which we methylate our DNA, how our Methylation Cycle functions and is impacted by diet and toxins alters not only our health but the health of our descendants. **When I say that thinking about the Methylation Cycle**

is something we all need to be concerned about, I truly mean <u>all</u> of us.

Environmental toxins also have the capacity to negatively influence methylation. Such that your diet, exposure to toxins, as well as your genetics and inherited epigenetics all play a role in your susceptibility to health conditions. Toxins create a catch 22, as they impair methylation and the degree of DNA methylation in turn plays a role in your susceptibility to environmental toxins. This again emphasizes that there are a number of factors that come into play to create a perfect storm of nonideal health.

It is not just about the car you were given in this life. It is also about the way you drive that car, how well your personal mechanic for that car functions and the type of fuel and environmental elements that car is exposed to that determine how long and how well your car will survive. Your car for life is your DNA. Your mechanic for life is your epigenetics. If your mechanic is nonfunctional, then no matter how lovely a car you were given at birth and no matter how carefully you drive and maintain that car it is going to slowly accumulate mechanical issues over time without a mechanic. On the other hand, if your car is well maintained with regular visits to your personal mechanic, then even if your car has some weaknesses it can last a lifetime.

CHAPTER 12

Following the Map Through the Short Cut

After looking at thousands of SNP results for the Methylation Cycle, there are some combinations of mutations that I have never seen. These would be combinations that completely disable the Methylation Cycle to the point where it is nonfunctional. For this reason I believe that a functional Methylation Cycle is a necessary condition for survival. **In my personal opinion, if the mythical fountain of youth did exist, it would in fact be the Methylation Cycle.** This cycle has the capacity to impact miscarriages, neural tube defects, cancer, heart disease, stroke, Alzheimer's, depression, anemia and even gray hair or the ability to wake up after anesthesia. This set of traffic circles that affects the entire *circle of life*, from pregnancy to old age is clearly a pathway worth getting in balance.

There are two routes around the methionine/folate cycles; in other words two ways to get around the first two traffic circles.

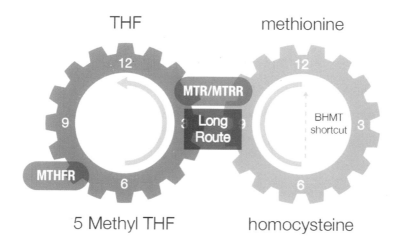

The ultimate goal is to traverse the "long route" around the first two traffic circles through the juncture where B12 sits, however this can cause excretion of toxins from the body. While detoxification is a good thing, it can also allow for symptoms during the detoxification process. It is possible to just get this critical cycle moving by supporting the "short cut" to restore methylation function while limiting potential detoxification reactions. The "short cut" is a direct route from homocysteine to methione. This short cut does not go through the juncture where B12 plays a role. It is just a quick trip from homocysteine directly to methioinine thus helping to ensure homocysteine does not climb too high while allowing methionine to increase. There are supplements that can help to support this short cut including a mixture of compounds called "phospholipids" and specific types of oils. The use of particular molecules including docosahexaenoic acid (DHA), phosphatidylserine (PS), phosphatidylcholine (PC), phosphatidylethanolamine (PE) and phosphatidylinositol (PI) can help to allow the short cut to function. These are long names of important compounds that will jump start your Methylation Cycle. The abbreviations PS, PC, PE, PI along with DHA make it easier to remember which nutrients can help to ensure that you have at least some Methylation Cycle function even if you have a number of mutations in this pathway.

Many adults who have had SNPs in this pathway since birth, have very likely experienced a gradual depletion of Methylation Cycle function as there has been no support to bypass these mutations over the course of their lifetime. This is compounded by the fact that some of the players in these traffic circles lose activity with age. Thus aging itself allows for a natural depletion of Methylation Cycle function. If we combine aging, with mutations in this pathway, and infectious agents that impair these traffic circles and toxic metal accumulation...you can start to see why over time there is a decrease in health and well-being if you are not supporting the Methylation Cycle. I am not suggesting that nutritional support for the Methylation Cycle will prevent cancer, Alzheimer's disease, Parkinson's, stroke, heart attack, neural tube defects, miscarriages or gray hair. I am saying that by supporting this critical pathway in the body that you at least lower the risk due to a lack of Methylation Cycle function. I again repeat, there are some combinations of mutations that I have not seen, which would suggest the critical nature of this set of traffic circles in the body. The implication is that supporting this pathway may be one of the healthiest choices you can make for yourself and your family.

Getting some support for the short cut around the cycle is one way to jumpstart the Methylation Cycle. Long route support involves B12 support. In the past I felt that the more B12 you added the better. However, over time and experience I have qualified that statement. Research suggests that lithium, a mineral, plays a role in B12 transport. What I have found repeatedly on mineral testing is that a majority of those with a range of health issues are low in lithium. Adding B12 before lithium is in balance may cause further depletion of lithium.

CHAPTER 13

Keeping Track of Lithium

At this point I feel that keeping an eye on lithium levels, particularly for anyone adding any form of B12 is critical. At this time no one else is talking about the critical role of lithium with respect to B12. We all recognize the importance of B12 but we also need to be aware that if you are adding B12 you really want to pay attention to lithium levels and to be sure you are not depleting your system of lithium.

I believe that the role of lithium and the importance of lithium with regard to the Methylation Cycle has been under recognized and overlooked for a very long time. This is true with respect to both the adults on this program as well as individuals with autism.

As I have cited in the past, lithium is reported to play a role in the transport of B12. This would fit with the data I have accumulated which indicates that until lithium is in balance on a HMT (hair metal test) that the cobalt (a measure of B12) generally will not increase on a UEE (urine essential element test). In cases where blood B12 is high, yet urine cobalt is low we again see confirmation of the role of lithium, as in these cases the HMT lithium as well as blood lithium tends to be low. Once lithium is supported the B12 levels will also reach a better balance. The positive role of lithium is not limited to its impact on B12 transport.

Lithium is not only a factor in B12 transport, it has a range of other roles in the body. Lithium is well known to play a role in mood, and limiting aggression. It also helps in controlling excess glutamate in the system as well as its involvement in B12 transport.   Lithium has been reported to increase human gray matter in the brain (Moore, The Lancet). *"Defined human lithium deficiency diseases have not been observed. However, inverse associations of tap water lithium contents in areas of Texas with the rates of mental hospital admissions, suicides, homicides and certain other crimes suggest that low lithium intakes cause behavioral defects"* (Schrauzer, J Am Coll Nutr). This is supported by animal studies illustrating that lithium deficient rats showed behavioral abnormalities.   In these studies lithium has also been shown to impact fetal growth and development, with significant effects on birth rate, litter size and higher incidences of spontaneous miscarriages. Lithium reaches a maximum level during the first trimester, aiding in the expansion of the stem cell pool and impacting embryonic development. In addition, data indicates that those with Lyme disease are also low in lithium and that the use of lithium may be a help for this condition (Top Ten Lyme Disease Treatments, Rossner). In addition to its positive impact on gray matter, lithium also *"selectively increases neuronal differentiation of hippocampal neural progenitor cells both in vitro and in vivo"* (Kim, Journal of Neurochemistry).

Data from the American College of Nutrition suggests that 83% of our population is lithium deficient and recommend a *minimum* daily intake of at least 1mg/day (Journal of the American College of Nutrition). My personal opinion in terms of dosing, as with other supplements for this program, is that I rely strongly on biochemical data. I believe in regular testing, especially for those who have shown low in lithium or those who have a particular SNP in the MTR (methionine synthase) gene. In general for those where lithium is a significant issue I would run a HMT every three to four months. In addition, blood lithium tests can also be run to supplement hair data. Estimates of the ideal average intake and recommended dose for lithium range from 650 to 3100 micrograms for a 70 kg adult (Schrauzer, J Am Coll Nutr) to therapeutic doses that are approximately ten times higher. *"Since Lithium is minimally protein bound and has an apparent volume of distribution of 0.6 L/kg. The therapeutic dose is 300–2700 mg/d"* (Mohandas Indian J Psychiatry). Daily increases of only 0.4 milligrams of dietary lithium have been sufficient in some cases to demonstrate improvements in cognitive function as well as mood

(Schrauzer, Biological Trace Element Research). **As always, with any supplementation, work with and defer to your own doctor in terms of use and dosage.**

The goal is to be certain lithium is in balance without levels becoming too high. The best way to ensure balance in my personal opinion is to run frequent HMT, blood tests if needed and as always work with and defer to your doctor. In my experience there is no perfect dose of lithium. Those who are on thyroid medication or taking iodine in higher doses may require more lithium as iodine will compete with lithium. Those who are using massive doses of B12 injections may require more lithium to keep it in balance (again as judged by biochemical testing). Those who have specific types of MTR mutations tend to have intrinsically lower lithium levels. I have a great deal of data supporting the fact that specific MTR (methionine synthase) SNPs correlate with low HMT lithium. As to why, I can hypothesize but this is an area where there is very little direct research on the interaction between B12 and lithium. Presumably this relationship is due to over activity of the MTR enzyme secondary to particular SNPs. Since MTR uses B12 and lithium plays a role in B12 transport you can see why it fits with the data that those who have particular MTR mutations that cause excess MTR activity would tend to require more lithium.

Again, to reiterate on lithium dosing…run tests on a regular basis! The goal is to keep lithium in balance without having it climb too high or be way too low. If you are supplementing with lithium and are seeing high level excretion in urine and hair then run a blood lithium test to determine if much of what you are supplementing with is simply being excreted. If you are supporting with lithium and your HMT gets into balance then run regular HMT to be sure that lithium at that dose stays in balance. I have noted that individuals with particular SNPs in the Methylation Cycle, such as a particular MTR mutation, tend to be very low in lithium as judged by hair metal analysis (HMT). For those with these specific MTR SNPs, the more B12 you add the more lithium may be needed, so again, run tests and as always work with your doctor. I have seen some unique cases where individuals were unable to keep lithium in balance using nutritional supplement sources of lithium. In these instances the use of prescription lithium was needed through consultation with their doctors.

Again, to reiterate one more time, it is my personal opinion and based on the data I have been generating, that lithium support is a critical missing piece of many supplement programs particularly for those using high dose B12. In order to be sure that lithium stays in balance, run frequent HMT and if needed blood lithium levels. **As always work with and defer to your own doctor.** Supporting with higher levels of B12 before having ascertained that lithium is in balance may lead to further depletion of lithium levels. For this reason I highly suggest running a hair metal test (HMT), and/or blood lithium test along with a urine essential element test (UEE) to assess the lithium level in the system BEFORE looking to add long route support. If lithium levels are low in hair and blood or urine, or if very high level lithium excretion is observed (in the absence of support) consider additional lithium supplementation with your doctor before moving on to B12 support.

Finally, there is a close relationship between lithium levels in hair and potassium levels. Potassium is critical for muscle function, and lack of potassium can also play a role in aggressive behavior (along with low lithium). **It is my personal opinion that potassium support should always be considered when supporting with lithium.** Again, as always work with and defer to your own doctor in terms of any supplementation program.

CHAPTER 14

Determine Your Ideal Form of B12

Once your lithium levels are in balance and short cut support is in place it is time to start to increase B12 support and to customize your supplement plan to optimize your health. Vitamin B12 is a water soluble vitamin. This means that it doesn't stay in the body for a long period of time and that more frequent support with B12 may be needed to maintain healthy B12 levels in the body. This means that as you add more B12 you want to pay attention to lithium levels so that the ideal balance exists between much needed B12 support and being sure that lithium is not depleted in the process. (In addition, as you support with lithium, also pay careful attention that potassium stays in balance and consider potassium support when adding lithium). Vitamin B12 not only plays a crucial role in the long route around the cycle it is a critical B vitamin with a wide range of roles in the body.

Vitamin B12 is important for energy, for balance related sports and for endurance sports. B12 is needed for healthy red blood cells, and for memory. Vitamin B12 can be depleted by drinking alcoholic beverages, a poor diet, certain medications and as we age. Vegetarians are often deficient in B12 as red meat is a major source of B12. Lack of B12 has been associated with fatigue, alcoholic liver disease, anemia, cancer, ulcers, dementia, neural tube defects, depression and memory loss. Higher levels of B12 correlate with improved balance, energy and endurance in athletics.

Different types of B12 work best for different people.

Just as the GPS system in your car guides you in unknown areas when you are driving, so too can your nutrigenomic results guide you in individualizing your personal healthcare. Not all of us can tolerate caffeine. We all know people who can drink espresso just before bed and fall asleep like a baby and others who are shaking from a single cup of dilute coffee. These differences in part reflect individual tolerances to certain compounds in coffee. These effects are similar to the response people can have to different forms of B12.

Vitamin B12, also called cobalamin, can include hydroxyl B12, methyl B12, cyano B12 and adenosyl B12. Many vitamins, including B12, are not active in the form in which they are normally found in food, instead the body needs to convert the B12 into a form that it can use directly. B12 is needed for the proper functioning of a number of different enzymes in the body;

however not all types of B12 are equal and not all types of B12 can be easily changed to what is needed for critical reactions in the body. Hydroxy, methyl and adenosyl are all forms of B12 that are used directly for reactions in the body. CyanoB12 must be converted for use in the body and as the name suggests, CyanoB12 or cyanocobalamin contains a cyanide molecule.

- MethylB12 can be used in the body, though it cannot be tolerated by everyone. Those who get jittery from caffeine, coke, tea may not react as well to methylB12. Many adults don't do as well with methyl B12 in spite of their nutrigenomics and so it is fine to choose an alternative form.

- AdenosylB12 is a special form of B12 that is important in the energy cycle in the cells of your body. It is important to have adenosyl B12 but it is not as versatile as other forms of B12 so it can be used in lower doses.

- Hydroxycobalamin, or hydroxyB12 is a unique form of vitamin B12, which is more easily converted to the form that is actually used for reactions in the body. This might cause you to ask, why doesn't everyone use high dose hydroxylB12 in their formulations? Well, Hydroxycobalamin (Hydroxy B12) is more difficult to work with, harder to keep in an active form and more expensive than some other forms of B12, such as cyanoB12. For this reason, many other products do not contain hydroxyl B12 and instead use cyanoB12.

• CyanoB12 contains a cyanide molecule. So when you take cyanoB12 your body must first convert it to hydroxyB12 in order to use it, and then must find a way to get rid of the toxic cyanide molecule. We all know cyanide is a poison even if the rest of the B12 molecule is good for you. The body actually uses hydroxyB12 in order to detoxify cyanide. So, not only is cyanoB12 not the form your body ultimately needs, but taking higher doses of cyanoB12 may actually deplete your hydroxy B12. So why would anyone use cyano B12 if it can be toxic? For the most part cyanoB12 is used because it is much less expensive, and a form of B12 that is easier to keep stable.

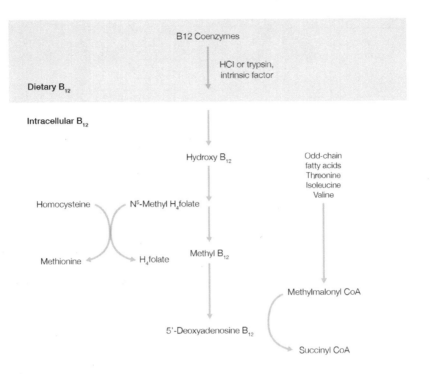

FIGURE 27.14
Metabolism of vitamin B12.
The metabolic interconversions of B12 are indicated with black arrows, and B_{12}-requiring reactions are indicated with red arrows. Other related pathways are indicated with blue arrows.

Devlin, T. 2002 Biochemistry with Clinical Correlations Wiley and Sons

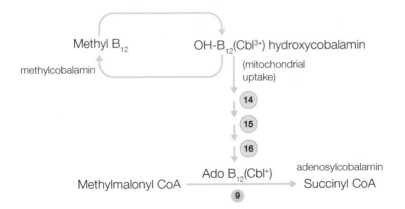

Basic Neurochemistry Molecular, Cellular and Medical Aspects George J. Siegel M.D., et al

Symptoms of lack of B12

Apathy

Drowsiness

Restlessness

Indifference to surroundings

Emotional instability

Loss of inhibition

Gradual mental deterioration

Delerium

Apprehension

Neurasthenia

Hysteria

Violent outbursts

Epilepsy

Confusion

Hallucinations

Delusions

Disorientation

Confabulation

Anxiety

Fatigue

Depression

Irritability

Sleepiness

Psychosis

Introspection

Stupor

Slow cerebration

Lack of energy

Weakness

Subacute organic reactions

Self pity

Flight of ideas

Negativism

Acute paranoia

Insomnia

Apprehensiveness

Memory impairment

Paraphrenia

Panic attacks

Dementia praecox

CHAPTER 15

Working on the Long Route

In addition to the use of Vitamin B12, support for the long route around the cycle also uses folate. Those with MTHFR (methyl tetra hydrofolate) mutations cannot use plain folate directly and instead use a special form of folate called 5 methyl THF which helps to bypass these MTHFR mutations.

If possible I would suggest a source of 5 methyl THF that gives you control over dosing such that you can adjust the dose down to a very low level. This is important as the addition of 5 methylTHF will often be the piece that triggers significant excretion of toxic substances from the body. Having the ability to adjust this process is a real plus as it allows you to limit the dose of 5 methylTHF and hence to have some control over the rate of detoxification. In general I prefer to use smaller amounts of a range of supplements and herbs to support the system naturally.

I am well aware that there are other programs that use much higher doses of 5 methyl THF. While this is not my preference at all, you can increase the amount of 5 methyl THF as needed to adapt to whatever program you are using. I see the Roadmap to health as a marathon, not a sprint. A change in the way you approach life, look at health and supporting your body. This program is not a quick fix high dose solution. Rather than approaching healthcare as something to rush through and just get finished with, I use a different lens or vantage point to approach personal healthcare. You are going to care about your health more than almost anyone else. You have the capacity to take charge of your own health with this program. You have the ability to make balancing the Methylation Cycle just another part of your daily routine.

The use of 5 formyl THF (this is a different molecule and a different supplement than 5 methyl THF) will feed directly into the points of the pathway that synthesize the DNA and RNA bases, known as nucleotides. DNA and RNA are critical for new cell synthesis and cellular repair. Due to the essential role that these nucleic acids and their building blocks serve in the body it is wise to supplement these compounds in a redundant fashion. In addition to the use of 5 formyl THF, I suggest that you directly add nucleotides to take some strain off of the pathway. Supplementation with specific RNAs may also be beneficial in terms of adding more complete RNA molecules so that the pathway does not need work to produce RNA sequences under conditions where the body is lacking components of the required pathway for these essential molecules.

Support for the secondary pathway, the "short cut" through the cycle can also take some of the burden off the "long route" around the cycle. The idea is to continue to support the path going from homocysteine directly to methionine, the short cut, while simultaneously supplementing the long route via methionine synthase (MTR) and methionine synthase reductase (MTRR).

Small amounts of plain methionine can also be used and, if indicated by genetics, the addition of SAMe (s adenosyl methionine) help to support at additional steps of these cycles. **SAMe is often referred to as the universal methyl donor, as it provides the methyl groups for DNA, RNA, histones, neurotransmitters, membrane phospholipids, proteins, melatonin and numerous small molecules.**

The goal is to use low doses of a variety of supplements to support a number of points of the pathway. I have found that this is easier on the system than using high doses of just a few supplements for this pathway. One way to understand this concept is to think of mutations in the pathway as accidents on a roadway. While it is possible to use a bulldozer to clear an accident that approach causes a great deal of collateral damage. On the other hand, if you recognize that there is more than one way to get from point A to point B, that you can take the highway, a second major roadway, a side road and a number of back roads, this opens up more gentle approaches to addressing the "accident" on the freeway. If you look to clear or bypass the accident as well as ensuring that all of the alternate routes are supported properly then you are more likely to keep traffic flowing in spite of the blockade on your major highway. The philosophy here is to recognize the pathways involved, the way in which they are interconnected and then supplement with small amounts of a number of nutrients to support the overall health of the entire pathway.

It is important to keep in mind as you begin to supplement or bypass your genetic weaknesses in this pathway, that this pathway is also involved in the ability to silence viral infections and to detoxify environmental toxins and heavy metals. As you support this pathway, so that it functions properly, perhaps for the first time in your life, it may help your body to trigger natural detoxification mechanisms. While detoxification is important for overall long term health and wellness there can be temporary discomforts associated with the detoxification process. This is another reason to use the more gentle approach of supplementing with low doses of a number of supplements, rather than using the bulldozer (high dose) approach. There are simple noninvasive tests that can be utilized to monitor the rate of excretion of toxins from your system as you support your body to bypass Methylation Cycle mutations. As you detoxify you begin to lower the impact of environmental risk factors that affect your long term health and wellness.

CHAPTER 16

Detours and Exit Ramps

Aside from MTHFR mutations here are a number of other SNPs that impact the flow of traffic through the traffic circles that make up the Methylation Cycle. The SHMT (serine hydroxy methyl transferase) SNP is like a detour to nowhere that diverts traffic from your Methylation Cycle. There is a purpose to the SHMT detour and that is to produce certain building blocks for your DNA and for your immune system. It is possible to simply add these building blocks to support your immune system and new DNA synthesis. This decreases the need for the detour to siphon off your Methylation Cycle intermediates and allows more of the supplements you are adding to remain in the set of four traffic circles that make up the Methylation Cycle.

A second key mutation that has the capacity to divert compounds from your Methylation Cycle are certain types of CBS (cystathionine beta synthase) SNPs. The CBS path is like an exit ramp out of the traffic circle that does not allow the traffic to reenter the Methylation Cycle. Some CBS mutations block this ramp, other types of CBS mutations divert a majority of the traffic flow through this exit ramp. The nutrigenomic test that I utilize looks only at those CBS mutations that divert traffic via this exit ramp, out of the critical Methylation Cycle traffic circles. Even if you have not run this particular nutrigenomic test, **those with this type of CBS mutation will tend toward excessively high taurine levels on a urine amino acid (UAA) test once methylation support is in place. Until adequate support for the Methylation Cycle is in place the impact of the CBS SNP is often not seen.**

Another way to think of the CBS mutations that force you to exit the highway with no path to reentry is as a leaky plug in a bath tub. Until you fill the tub with water you cannot tell that the drain plug isn't sealing properly and is causing the tub water to flow down the drain instead of filling the tub. In a similar fashion, you cannot see the impact of the CBS SNP until you have sufficient methylation support in place such that the cycle is filling and at that point the taurine levels will rise well above the 50th percentile on a UAA. Work with your doctor to use UAA testing to monitor taurine levels. Once taurine levels do climb, work in conjunction with your doctor to add supports as needed to keep taurine in balance and use consistent UAA testing to track taurine levels.

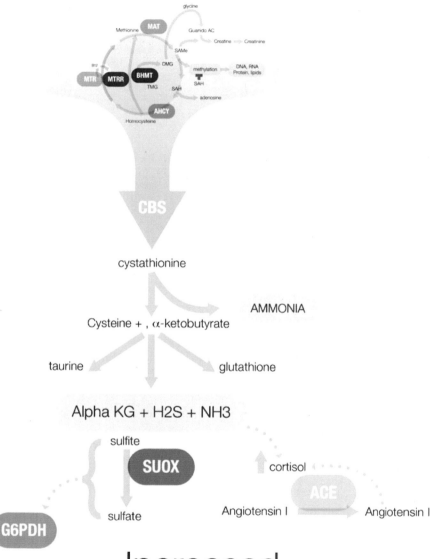

Increased
CBS Enzyme Activity

CHAPTER 17

Signposts Along the Way

While your epigenetics are influenced by diet, toxins and heredity, your DNA does not change. Nutrigenomic SNP testing is something you will run only once in your lifetime. Unlike DNA based SNP testing, follow up biochemical testing is something you can run routinely to check that the supplementation you are using is actually making a difference.

I view biochemical tests like signs along a highway that let you know where you are located in your journey and how much further you need to go to reach your destination. I often have individuals who have run a nutrigenomic test to see where the imbalances are in their Methylation Cycle. They then add what appears to be appropriate supplementation based on those nutrigenomic results to support the short cut and the long route around the cycle. I will get a question on the discussion group about what they should add next. My question back to them is always what are your biochemical tests looking like? Asking what to do next without running biochemical tests is like calling on your way from your hometown to my rural town in Maine.

How can you ask which route to take, if you cannot answer where you are located? How can you ask how much longer the trip will take, if you don't know where you are on the Roadmap?

This program can help you to plot your Roadmap to health, but you need to have a sense of where you are on the road in order to know the next step to take.

Starting with nutrigenomic testing is a wonderful place to begin as it is possible to look at specific supplementation to bypass mutations that are identified by SNP testing. But the next critical piece is to be sure you are running biochemical tests to be sure the support you are adding is sufficient and having the impact you desire. Biochemical tests are like signposts along the highway on your Roadmap to Health. While you can get started on your journey without nutrigenomic testing, it is virtually impossible to know where you are on the path to health without running biochemical tests.

The tests I work from are noninvasive in nature that can be run from the privacy of your own home. I find that there is much better compliance when you have control over when and where you take a test. You can also run additional blood tests with your own doctor to supplement the results from urine, hair and fecal testing.

Urine amino amino tests give you information about the building blocks for proteins in your system. UAA testing can help you to see if you are making progress with some of the compounds in the Methylation Cycle as well as a sense of overall nutrient absorption. UAA tests measure homocysteine which is a compound associated with a range of health imbalances, as well as methionine,taurine and phospholipids which are all indicators of Methylation Cycle support.

Urine essential and toxic elements tests (UTM/UEE) give you a picture of the toxins being excreted from your system as well as the level of critical minerals in your body. Toxic metal excretion data is useful as the environmental toxic load can impair methylation and also is one of the risk factors in multifactorial conditions. Cobalt levels on an essential mineral test can give indicators about Methylation Cycle support as cobalt is a measure of B12 levels. Where lithium is reported to impact B12 transport having data on lithium levels in urine as well as hair can be a help in supporting the Methylation Cycle.

Hair metal tests give additional information about toxic and essential mineral levels. HMT are particularly useful with respect to lithium levels. Research suggests that hair tests are an excellent measure of lithium levels. Blood lithium testing can also be run. When adding Vitamin B12 to support the Methylation Cycle I feel it is critical to closely follow lithium levels (as well as potassium).

Metabolic Analysis testing helps to give information about intermediates in the Methylation Cycle, about breakdown products of neurotransmitters like serotonin and dopamine and also gives data concerning critical energy intermediates in the body. More and more adults and children are recognizing mitochondrial issues as a factor in their declining health. MAP testing is useful in assessing the level of mitochondrial energy intermediates.

Another key factor in multifactorial conditions is the infectious disease burden. In addition to blood testing for antibody titers for a range of bacterial and viral conditions, there are stool tests that can be utilized. Comprehensive stool analysis tests and DNA probe tests can give an indication of the bacterial and yeast load in the intestinal tract. I like to run both tests simultaneously as they give related but nonidentical information. The comprehensive stool analysis does not limit the organisms it allows to grow but will indicate any organisms that are present that grow in a given amount of time. This is a wonderful tool to see the range of nonideal organisms in the gut. But a comprehensive stool analysis may not pick up very slow growing or oxygen sensitive organisms. Tests that use a DNA based probe often detect very small numbers of slow growing organisms. This is excellent for determining if slow growing organisms are an issue even if they did not grow on the comprehensive stool analysis. However, DNA probe tests only look for a limited number of organisms so it can only identify those for which the DNA probe is included in the test. For this reason the combination of a comprehensive stool analysis along with DNA probe based tests for microorganisms yield more comprehensive data in my opinion.

Again, the purpose of biochemical tests is to follow up on the supplementation you are using based on nutrigenomic testing. If you have not run a nutrigenomic test you can still get a sense of where you are on your Roadmap to health by running biochemical tests. The nutrigenomic SNP testing gives you an idea about underlying genetic weaknesses. The biochemical tests give you feedback on how well your current support regime is working so you can determine where you are located on your personal Roadmap to health and wellness.

CHAPTER 18

Infectious Burdens

Scientifically, we are just beginning to understand that health issues do not occur as an isolated incident or event in the absence of other contributing factors. Many different factors act together to influence the development of health problems. Variables like age and gender along with other genetic and environmental factors may play a role in the onset of **multifactorial conditions**.

Rather than a simple case of using an antibiotic for a bacterial infection or a vaccine to prevent a viral infection or the one gene/one disease theory, the story is more complex. The infectious disease landscape itself has also become more complicated in spite of the advent of antibiotics and more aggressive vaccination programs since the 1950's. Not only are our tools to deal with health conditions more sophisticated today but also the diseases themselves and the advent of multiple antibiotic resistant organisms emphasize that this is not as simplistic as we first perceived it to be in the 1950's.

We now talk in terms of the "total microbial or pathogen burden", and its effect upon an individual. It is not uncommon in this day and age for people to harbor a number of chronic bacterial and viral infections in their system simultaneously. These organisms can be seen as taking advantage of an unhealthy body to set up housekeeping in a system that has the right conditions to allow them to grow and flourish.

The issue is not just the microbial organism per se, rather multisystem imbalances in the body that create an atmosphere that allows for the growth of these opportunistic organisms. **Recognize that you need to address the microbial environment as well as the specific offending microbes**. Simply put, if your gut is a swamp you are going to attract offensive organisms as compared to a more pristine gastrointestinal environment.

This is not that dissimilar from termites infesting rotting wood. While this is a repulsive visual image, it makes the point that it is important to look at all aspects that affect health in your life, to prevent your body from becoming a veritable pillar of rotting wood that will allow the growth of the microbiological equivalent of termites in your system.

A slightly less distasteful way to look at "opportunistic" organisms is to think of them in terms of their ability to take advantage of you. Opportunistic organisms are not unlike invaders in your home. Opportunistic organisms invade your body when it is vulnerable in the same way that an intruder will invade your home if it is unlocked with the front door left wide open! While it is still possible to have an intruder even with the best security precautions, you are less likely to have intruders if the front door is closed and locked. In a similar manner you may sometimes become ill even if you take excellent care of your body. However, we can reduce the risk of human invasion into our homes with proper prevention, just as we can reduce the risk of opportunistic microbial invasion in our bodies with proper attention to all aspects of our health.

Supporting with a range of specific normal flora may help to populate the gut with preferred species and serve as a protective layer from nonideal organisms. Realize that your intestinal tract houses up to 100 trillion microbes. Helping to define those organisms aids in creating a positive gut environment, one that is less conducive to the growth of disease causing bacteria.

You can think of the lining of your gut as a brick wall. Assume for this example that the bricks are not held together with mortar. Like a well-built brick wall, this wall will withstand the test of time without mortar to hold the bricks together if you choose the building materials wisely. On the other hand, if the bricks don't fit together well, if there are huge gaps between them, then water, mold and debris will begin to accumulate in those gaps. Over time the wall will begin to slowly decay as the integrity has been impaired. So too, if your gut is not lined with healthy normal flora it opens the door for less desired bacteria to inhabit the area. The gaps in the wall of normal flora allow for leakage of food particles through the gut wall, which can be a factor in allergic and inflammatory gut conditions.

"The adult human intestine is home to an almost inconceivable number of microorganisms. The size of the population— up to 100 trillion—far exceeds that of all other microbial communities associated with the body's surfaces and is ... Thus, it seems appropriate to view ourselves as a composite of many species and our genetic landscape as an amalgam of genes embedded in our Homo sapiens genome and in the genomes of our affiliated microbial partners (the microbiome)...The gut microbiome, which may contain > 100 times the number of genes in our genome, endows us with functional features that we have not had to evolve ourselves" (Backhed, Science).

My personal preference for probiotics is a mixture of normal flora that is focused on species of *Lactobacillus* and *Bifidobacter* as the main sources of normal flora. I have found that this helps to create a gut environment that is less likely to allow for the growth of nonideal microbes.

Normal flora helps to protect the gut from the growth of pathogenic organisms. Antibiotic use is well known to cause imbalances in normal gut flora. The use of antibiotics without concurrent addition of probiotics, therefore, can predispose to the growth of streptococci as well as other pathogenic organisms.

Unfortunately many individuals have issues with chronic streptococcal infection or chronic issues with other bacteria in the body. Streptococcal infection in the gut can serve as a reservoir to reinfect the sinuses. Chronic streptococcal infection has been associated with OCD behavior as well as tics, over stimulatory behavior and perseverative speech. Streptococcal infection can also lay the groundwork for leaky gut which can relate to decreased weight gain or slower growth.

"Imbalances in the flora of the GI tract may begin as early as birth. Maternal streptococci, for example, can be transmitted from the mother to the neonate during delivery. Although researchers originally believed that transmission occurred solely via vaginal delivery, more recent data suggest that streptococcal infection can also occur in infants who have been delivered via cesarean section. The rate of mother-to-infant transmission of streptococci during vaginal delivery is between 20 and 30 percent" (Yasko and Mullan, Autism Science Digest).

Studies have shown that there is an interaction between the immune system, the nervous system, and the microbial environment within the gut. In this way, gastrointestinal function not only affects digestion but also the function of other organs and systems in the body, most notably the brain and nervous system.

"Over the past few decades, research has significantly changed the way that scientists understand gastrointestinal (GI) function and dysfunction. We have come to recognize that the GI tract is, in fact, far more subtle and complex than initially thought. Studies have illuminated how the complex interaction of the immune system, the neuroendocrine system, and the microbial environment within the gut affects not only GI function but also the function of other organs and systems in the body, most notably the brain and nervous system. We now understand that body systems and organs function within a web of physiology and biochemistry, and we no longer consider each system as discrete and isolated from the others" (Yasko and Mullan, Autism Science Digest).

Infection with a particular type of streptococcus, *group A beta-hemolytic Streptococcus* can result in a pediatric syndrome labeled pediatric autoimmune neuropsychiatric disorders (PANDAS). Individuals with PANDAS develop tics, OCD symptoms, and, in some cases, psychosis.

Chronic streptococcal infection, and possibly *Escherichia coli* infection can lead to a variety of inflammatory mediators as well as depleting neurotransmitters. Streptococcal infection leads to elevated levels of the inflammatory mediators that have been directly implicated in Tourette syndrome, facial tics, OCD behavior, and schizophrenia. These same inflammatory mediators can also allow for elevated levels of glutamate, an excitotoxin; excess excitotoxins can excite nerves to death.

Lack of Vitamin B12 is well documented to cause a range of neurological symptoms. There is a close relationship between gut health and vitamin B12 levels. One of the factors that contribute to increased gut acidity and gut flora imbalances include vitamin B12 deficiency. Excess stomach acid in the system can cause loose stools and severe stomach pain, increased gut acidity also can predispose to microbial imbalance. This deficiency in B12 can stem from particular Methylation Cycle SNPs or the presence of *Helicobacter pylori*, the bacterium that causes stomach ulcers. In addition, the use of antacids and medications for acid reflux can also decrease B12 levels. Intrinsic factor is a substance produced by the gastric lining that helps the body to absorb vitamin B12. Sufficient stomach acid is necessary for intrinsic factor activation. Efforts by the body to increase B12 levels lead to increased intrinsic factor and would be expected to increase stomach acid. Thus, Methylation Cycle SNPs that decrease the level of B12 in the body can contribute to an environment that is conducive to the growth of microbes that can flourish in an acidic environment.

While the growth of many bacteria is inhibited in an acidic environment, several bacteria can survive and flourish in a more acidic environment including *Streptococcus* (the bacteria that is a culprit in strep throat), *Escherichia coli* (the bacteria that can cause food poisoning and urinary tract infections) and *Helicobacter pylori* (the bacteria associated with stomach ulcers and cases of acid reflux). Increased stomach acid secondary to B12 deficiency, therefore, leads to a gut environment that predisposes to the growth pathogenic bacteria that can survive in an acid milieu. This is a key example of why you want to work on both the gut environment as well as the specific offending organisms. Until you change the environment you will continually battle the same nonideal organisms.

Helicobacter pylori itself has been reported to be a factor in B12 deficiency. This lack of B12 creates a catch 22, such that it contributes to the more acidic environment that can then attract the presence of *H. pylori* as well as other nonideal organisms.

Helicobacter pylori is an ulcer-causing gastric pathogen that is able to colonize the harsh acidic environment of the human stomach. Reportedly one third to half the adult population harbors *H. pylori* in their systems. Recent findings suggest that children with autism have a much higher than expected incidence of *H. pylori* (Yasko). Although the stomach is protected from its own gastric juice by a thick layer of mucus that covers the stomach lining, *H. pylori* takes advantage of this protection by living in the mucus lining itself. In the mucus lining, *H. pylori* survives the stomach's acidic conditions by producing ammonia. The ammonia creates a cloud around the bacterium, making it possible for *H. pylori* to escape the harsh acid environment. Because *H. pylori* burrows into the mucus layer of the stomach and is very persistent there, it is difficult to get a positive test for it when it is present and is extremely difficult to eradicate. *H. pylori* affects neurotransmitters and brain neurochemistry. *H. pylori* infection increases the incidence of food allergy by facilitating the passage of intact proteins across the gastric epithelial barrier. *H. pylori* also decreases levels of B12 in the body and increases ammonia which in turn can decrease BH4. *H. pylori* infection is not just an immediate acute infection. Rather, it is a long-term chronic problem that may take months or years to eradicate. Chronic *H. pylori* gastritis alters feeding behaviors, delays gastric emptying, alters gastric neuromuscular function, impairs acetylcholine release; these effects can persist for months after the infection has been eradicated.

Multiple factors impact the ability of bacteria to survive and flourish. In addition to taking advantage of an acidic environment, many microbes require the presence of iron for growth and/or virulence. Recall that iron also helps to cause a detour to nowhere described above in terms of the SHMT SNP in the Methylation Cycle. If addressing chronic microbial issues are goals of your personal Roadmap to health, then a strong consideration would be to use a general vitamin that is not high in iron.

As chronic bacterial infection is addressed it should help to aid in aluminum excretion since bacteria appear to retain and sequester aluminum. Aluminum is known to have a range of toxic effects in the body, including interfering with pathways that help to decrease excess glutamate. In addition, aluminum interferes with the production of BH4 regardless of the presence of specific MTHFR SNPs that negatively impact BH4 levels. Therefore, the presence of aluminum may be indirectly affecting levels of serotonin as well as dopamine in the body through its effects on BH4.

One of the overall impacts of chronic infection in the body is to increase oxidative stress and stimulate the immune system. Both of these factors can negatively influence BH4 which, again, can decrease the levels of your 'feel good' neurotransmitters, serotonin and dopamine.

A very high protein diet can also affect BH4 levels. Ammonia is generated from the intake of high protein foods. The body uses two molecules of BH4 to detoxify one molecule of ammonia to urea. This is an 'expensive' way to use your BH4. Again, recall that BH4 is also needed for dopamine and serotonin. This is just another example of looking at the multifactorial factors that come together to play a role in health. A high protein diet combined with chronic bacterial and viral issues that cause oxidative stress and immune activation, along with SNPs that decrease BH4 and aluminum retention by nonideal microbes...can all contribute to a perfect storm of complex health conditions

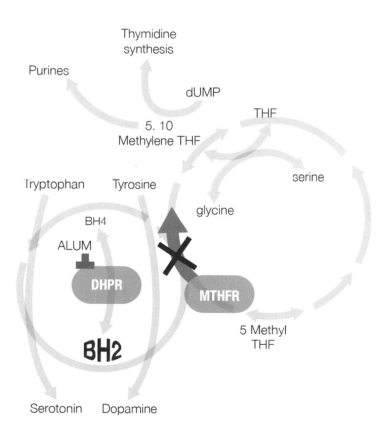

CHAPTER 19

Environmental Burdens

In the book, "The Puzzle of Autism: Putting It All Together" (Yasko) I presented the hypothesis that chronic viral and bacterial organisms in our bodies are able to create additional havoc in your system by acting as "accomplices" to heavy metals, and aiding in their retention in the body. This adds yet another layer of complication to the story and again reiterates the fact that the health conditions we face today are multifactorial and complex in nature.

While the bacteria staphylococci are especially prone to retaining aluminum, it is likely that other bacteria also can do so. Aluminum may increase the propensity for bacteria to form a biofilm, which is an additional survival mechanism used by bacteria to hide in the body in a chronic fashion. Bacterial infection promotes accumulation and retention of heavy metals in the body, which contributes to oxidative stress and impairs neurotransmitter formation. Metals may be retained in the body through several mechanisms.

The elimination of pathogenic gastrointestinal flora and excretion of the metals they retain, therefore, may be essential for proper function of the biochemical pathways in the body, along with maintenance of proper balance among the organisms that should be present in the gastrointestinal tract.

"Aluminum is a well-documented and undisputed neurotoxin that is associated with cognitive, psychological, and motor abnormalities. Both clinical observation and animal experiments have documented neurotoxicity from excess brain exposure to aluminum, which has been found in elevated levels in the brains of patients with Parkinsonism, amyotrophic lateral sclerosis (ALS), and Alzheimer-type dementia. Aluminum induces encephalopathy and causes neuroanatomical and neurochemical changes in the brain, including neurofilament disturbances followed by nerve cell loss. Primate studies have provided evidence of aluminum's ability to induce seizures" (Yasko and Mullan, Autism Science Digest).

In addition to aluminum toxicity, the presence of lead, arsenic, mercury and cadmium have been known to have adverse biological effects on humans since ancient times.   Metals, particularly heavy metals such as lead, cadmium and arsenic constitute significant potential threats to human health in both occupational and environmental settings. Arsenic is clearly carcinogenic and cadmium is now being recognized as a contributor to osteoporosis. Lead averages 1000 times higher concentration in all human bones tested anywhere on earth today than four centuries ago. During the past three decades epidemiologic studies have demonstrated inverse associations between blood lead concentrations and children's IQs at successively lower lead concentrations (Rogan, New England J Med). In response, the Center for Disease Control and Prevention (CDC) has repeatedly lowered its definition of an elevated blood lead concentration, which now stands at 10 µg per deciliter (0.483 µmol per liter). The fact that associations are seen at these low lead concentrations implies that there is no safe level of lead. Mercury is neurotoxic even at the relatively low levels of exposure seen in dentists' offices. Many vaccines continue to include mercury as an ingredient. Coal-fired power plants alone release over 50 tons of mercury into the air annually just from burning coal for our electric power (Johnson, Chem Eng News).

My experience has been that as infections are eliminated from the system we see a release of stored metals from the body. The success of this approach supports the premise that these chronic infections have been efficiently binding toxic metals in the body where no chelating agent (metal binding agent) seems to be able to effectively remove them. With the elimination of chronic bacteria, viruses and heavy metals, real improvements in health and wellness can be achieved.

CHAPTER 20

Methylation Sits at the Center of Multifactorial Conditions:

Why You Should be Concerned if Your Cycle is Not Working Properly

"Methylation happens over a billion times a second. It is like one big dance, with biochemicals passing methyl groups from one partner to another" (Braly, The H Factor Solution).

This is the most scientific chapter of this book and also one of the most important chapters. **Please take your time and slowly read through to understand how methylation impacts virtually every aspect of your health.** I want you to truly understand why methylation is so critical and why you should be concerned if you are not supporting this pathway in your body.

Methylation is central to such critical reactions in the body as:

- Repairing and building RNA and DNA
- Immune function (how your body responds to and fights infection)
- Digestive Issues
- DNA silencing
- Neurotransmitter balance
- Metal Detoxification

- Inflammation
- Membrane fluidity
- Energy production
- Protein activity
- Myelination
- Cancer prevention

Methylation is involved in almost every reaction in your body. Aside from its critical editing function, without proper methylation, there is increased vulnerability to viruses, impaired attention span, and less efficient nerve transmission and a greater predisposition to cancer.

For an organism to live, it must create new cells as fast as cells die. This requires that the body make millions of cells every minute, relying on DNA and RNA synthesis. DNA carries the blueprint, or genetic coding, needed to build the components of living organisms. Every time your body needs to repair the gut lining, or create an immune cell to respond to an immune threat, or to heal when you have cut yourself, you need to synthesize new DNA. But without a functioning methylation cycle, your DNA is not going to replicate properly. Mutations in the methylation pathway can cripple the ability of the body to make the building blocks needed for new DNA and RNA synthesis. Very similar to DNA is RNA, which is crucial to building proteins, transferring the information carried by your DNA and regulating your genes. In fact, RNA is even more abundant in your body than DNA. This reduced capacity for new DNA and RNA synthesis means that any new cell synthesis is impaired. A reduced synthesis capacity due to methylation cycle mutations is a particular issue for cells that already have difficulties meeting their needs for DNA and RNA synthesis under normal conditions. Problems in the methylation pathway limit nucleotide building blocks that the brain and other organs need for repair and growth. Bone marrow cells, lymphocytes, erythrocytes and some brain cells cannot make some of the DNA and RNA bases that they need for synthesis. Intestinal mucosa cells cannot make enough building blocks to fulfill the body's requirement for healthy gut. Stress increases the need for these building blocks to overcome negative effects of hormones released during stressful conditions. Cell repair after injury increases the need for nucleotide building blocks. The brain has the highest concentration of RNA in the body, and therefore has the highest requirement for RNA building blocks.

Universal lack of methylation and the inability to produce these building blocks for RNA synthesis also results in a situation where the body is lacking the required elements for specific genetic regulation. This regulation or silencing is a multistep process that involves RNA as well as methylation to be certain that only the desired genetic material is expressed.   As described earlier, epigenetics is the mechanism used by the body to turn on and off genes. It is the editing system that gives the body a second chance to get around direct mutations in our DNA. **Epigenetic modification of DNA occurs mainly on a very specific DNA building block called *cytosine*.** Cytosine is one of the four DNA bases found in organisms, including humans. It is one of the DNA building blocks that are produced by optimal functioning of the Methylation Cycle. So, take a moment and think about this...Methylation Cycle function is needed to produce the building blocks for DNA that are in turn the recipients of methylation groups in order to turn on and off that same DNA. You can start to see how intimately related your DNA synthesis and function is with respect to the Methylation Cycle. Methylation of these cytosine bases is generally correlated with silencing of genes.

Methylation is important for turning on and off mammalian DNA. This is true for silencing viral DNA in the body as well as cellular DNA. There are sections of the DNA that are regulatory regions, requiring methylation such that they turn on and off the information portions as they should. During development DNA methylation patterns are established and are essential for normal development. During new cell synthesis these patterns are then replicated. When these regions do not have the correct amount of methyl groups bound to them it can prevent the information from being turned off, resulting in autoimmunity, aging and cancer.

It has been estimated that 70 to 80% of the cytosine's found in particular patterns in the DNA are methylated in humans. The other 20% of these cytosine patterns that are not methylated are found in clusters known as "islands". These nonmethylated islands are most often found in the region that turns on the gene. Thus methylation of cytosines creates two distinct regions in the DNA, "unmethylated islands" and "methylated cytosine pattern sites" that are distributed throughout the genome. These methylated regions tend to be located at mutational hot spots; **one third of all single base mutations associated with cancer are at these sites.**

Methylation of cytosine also helps to maintain the large amount of the non-utilized portion of the human DNA in an inert state as well as helping to silence harmful DNAs. If you are short on methyl groups due to methylation cycle mutations then you will have less methyl groups for preventing autoimmunity and silencing genomes. This is true for silencing viral genomes as well as for regulating your own DNA. **The methylation process prevents the reading of inserted viral sequences**. One of the consequences of loss of methylation function is that it could cause the potentially harmful expression of these inserted viral genes. Under-methylation in normally silent regions of the DNA can cause the expression of inserted viral genes.

Certain disease states occur as a result of increases in the length of specific repeat sections in the genome. These special "repeat regions" are prior to the information or coding region of the DNA. These trinucleotide repeats are involved in certain disorders such as Friedreich's ataxia, Fragile X and Huntington's disease. When there is insufficient methylation capacity (mutations in the pathway) there is often not enough methyl groups to bind to these repeat regions, so they are able to multiply.   This results in very long repeat sections, much longer than they should be. **Studies have shown that inhibition of DNA methylation resulted in a 1000 fold increase in these three base repeat sections**. Therefore, decreased DNA methylation results in increases in trinucleotide repeats and increases the risks for these disorders. This creates a catch 22 as these long repeated sections then attract the limited methyl groups that are available. The consequent overmethylation of these repeat sections results in shutting off genes inappropriately.

Females contain two copies of the X chromosome. Silencing one of these two copies is essential for normal development. Methylation of the DNA is the mechanism by which the second X chromosome is silenced. The normally nonmethylated "islands" become methylated as part of this silencing process. A similar strategy is utilized to silence one of two copies of genes other than those on the X chromosome. In these cases the inactivated gene can be of either maternal or paternal origin. Loss of normal silencing as a result of decreased methylation contributes to a number of inherited diseases including Beckwith-Wiedemann, Prader-Willi and Angelman syndromes, among others.

The expression of many cellular genes is modulated by something called "histone acetylation" in addition to DNA methylation. Interestingly, methylation also plays a role in the histone acetylation process. Methylation also plays a pivotal role in establishing and maintaining an inactive state of a gene by rendering the chromatin structure inaccessible. **Methylation therefore plays an important role in development, imprinting, X-chromosome inactivation and tissue-specific gene expression**. Changes in DNA methylation profiles are common features of development and in a number of human diseases.

You can start to see how proper Methylation Cycle function would play a role in fetal development. It also plays a role in successful preconception supplementation to prevent miscarriages. Mutations in the MTHFR genes of the methylation pathway as well as mutations that lead to decreased B12 are risk factors for neural tube defects. Mutations in the methylation pathway, specifically certain MTR and MTRR SNPs, as well as elevated homocysteine are risk factors for having a child with Down's syndrome.

It is important to consider methylation pathway mutations when looking at supplementing with folate during pregnancy. One way to understand this more easily is to think about the studies on folate and neural tube defects. Using folate during pregnancy helps to decrease the risk of neural tube defects. This is not changing the DNA but having a regulatory effect on the ability of the DNA to be expressed, known as epigenetics. Now, if folate can make a difference in DNA expression, but you have a mutation so that you cannot use folate, then taking folate may not do any good; it is almost as if you never supplemented at all. Running a nutrigenomic test to determine the form of folate that will bypass mutations in your folate pathway will enable you to supplement with the appropriate form of folate and should help to reduce the risk of neural tube defects in a similar way to the use of plain folate in the absence of mutations in this pathway. The genetics of the parent are reflected in the child. So that if a pregnant mother has mutations that make her unable to utilize plain folate, you should consider testing the infant for similar weaknesses in this pathway. The sooner that you know if and where a newborn's genetic weaknesses reside in the methylation pathway the sooner you can start to supplement to bypass these mutations. Remember, by supplementing properly you should have the potential to bypass and compensate for the mutations. If this is commenced from day one you do not allow time for virus to build in the system (remember that methylation is necessary to silence virus). In addition, some of the mutations in the methylation cycle make it difficult to make new T cells which are a critical part of your immune system. This may make it easier for the immune system of infants to react to vaccines in the correct fashion. **If the methylation cycle is working properly from day one it should help with myelination, immune regulation and the ability to make new DNA and RNA that is needed for growing cells.**

In the methylation pathway, one crucial component for neurotransmitter balance is the component, S-adenosyl methionine, or SAMe (pronounced "sammy"). **SAMe is the most active methyl donor in your body, bringing methyl groups to numerous chemical compounds in your body**. It is a required participant in at least forty different critical reactions in the body. It also acts upon the neurotransmitters by changing them into other needed compounds. If we don't have sufficient SAMe—or if SAMe can't be recycled due to weaknesses in the methylation cycle, this can result in imbalances in our neurotransmitters, which in turn can impact mood, focus, sleep patterns, as well as a range of behaviors. The Methylation Cycle not only has to produce SAMe, it also has to recycle it.

Once SAMe has given up its methyl groups to help create neurotransmitters, it is then "recycled"—that is, re-methylated. After SAMe has received its new methyl groups, it can perform its job all over again. Because of its essential role in reactions involving neurotransmitters, it's not surprising that a lack of SAMe plays a role in neurodegenerative conditions. Due to Methylation Cycle weaknesses, some people can neither produce nor recycle SAMe. Furthermore, issues with the level of SAMe in the body became a larger problem as we age. Fortunately, we can supplement SAMe to bypass mutations and attain its many benefits.

Some specific reactions that involve SAMe include:

- Converting serotonin to melatonin which supports healthy sleep
- Glutathione synthesis which is critical for detoxification
- In the formation of myelin which surrounds and protects nerves
- To convert the neurotransmitter norepinephrine into epinephrine, (also known as adrenaline). Together norepinephrine and epinephrine regulate the fight-or-flight response and, along with dopamine, are critical for attention and focus.

- In the creation of CoQ10, creatine, and carnitine, compounds essential to the work of the mitochondria, the energy factories of our cells

Adequate levels of CoQ10 have also been identified as necessary nutrients to help prevent congestive heart failure. Clinically the supplement CoQ10 has been used in the treatment of angina, heart failure, prevention of reperfusion injury after coronary artery bypass and cardiomyopathy. The synthesis of CoQ10 in the body requires components of the Methylation Cycle; in particular it requires adequate levels of the compound SAMe (s adenosyl methionine) that is generated by the methylation cycle. Cholesterol lowering drugs (statin drugs) decrease the supply of CoQ10 in the body. **It may be particularly important for individuals taking statin drugs to be aware of the methylation status in their body and replenish CoQ10**. In addition, the relationship between elevated homocysteine levels, an increased risk of heart disease and the genetic risk associated with certain MTHFR mutations in the Methylation Cycle has been recognized for quite some time. Appropriate supplementation of the Methylation Cycle should be able to help compensate for this mutation.

The mitochondria are the energy producing organelles within each cell. Decreased mitochondrial energy has been implicated in chronic fatigue, fibromyalgia and mitochondrial disease. Coenzyme Q10 is also important for its role in energy production in the mitochondrial respiratory chain. Again, as mentioned above, Methylation Cycle function is necessary for the synthesis of CoQ10 in the body. Carnitine is another nutrient produced by the body that is involved in mitochondrial energy production. Mitochondria fatty acid oxidation is the main energy source for heart and skeletal muscle. Carnitine is also involved in the transport of these fatty acids into the mitochondrial matrix. As with CoQ10, the synthesis of carnitine by the body requires Methylation Cycle function. Synthesis of carnitine begins with methylation via the action of SAMe .**Low muscle tone and extreme muscle weakness may in part be due to decreased mitochondrial energy as well as myelination problems due to reduced Methylation Cycle capacity**. Methylation is also needed to produce creatine in the body. The methyl group for this reaction is again donated by SAMe. Creatine is a supplement taken by many weight lifters due to its role in muscle energy; creatine has also been reported to play a role in speech, language, attention span and ability to follow commands.

There is literature to suggest that ADD/ADHD can be helped by the addition of SAMe. SAMe is a critical intermediate in the Methylation Cycle. SAMe is also a methyl donor for reactions that involve dopamine, epinephrine and norepinephrine. Imbalances in this dopamine, epinephrine and norepinephrine have been implicated in ADD/ADHD. One can envision that Methylation Cycle function is needed to produce SAMe as a methyl donor for the dopamine/ nor epinephrine / epinephrine pathways to help to prevent ADD/ADHD. Impaired methylation results on a lack of components needed to generate feel good neurotransmitters like serotonin which regulates mood, emotion and appetite, as well as problems converting serotonin to melatonin so we can sleep at night. Many children with autism have difficulty sleeping as well as adults with chronic fatigue and fibromyalgia will frequently note sleep issues. Imbalances in methylation also affect dopamine levels as well as the dopamine receptor itself. Proper dopamine signaling requires that the dopamine receptor can move freely in the cell membrane. Methylation supports receptor activity by keeping the components of the cell membrane (phospholipids) more fluid. Imbalances in dopamine receptor signaling have been implicated in ADD/ADHD.

Myelin coating on nerves is important for proper neurotransmission. Myelin is a sheath that wraps around the neuronal wiring to insulate and facilitate faster transmission of electrical potentials. You can think of myelin as the coating around the electrical wires in your home. If those wires are not covered then even a single drop of water can cause the wire to short out. So too, your nerves are more vulnerable to assaults if they are not coated in myelin. **Without adequate methylation, the nerves cannot myelinate in the first place, nor remyelinate after insults such as viral infection or heavy metal toxicity**. In addition, methylation helps to stabilize myelin against degradation. Proper levels of methylation are also directly related to the body's ability to both myelinate nerves and to prune nerves. A secondary effect of a lack of methylation and hence decreased myelination is inadequate pruning of nerves. Pruning helps to prevent excessive wiring of unused neural connections and reduces the synaptic density. Without adequate pruning the brain cell connections are misdirected and proliferate into dense, bunched thickets. All of these changes, when they occur in utero or in very young children, can alter brain development and can also set up metabolic changes that cause ongoing compromise of brain function. These metabolically caused changes in brain function may, however, be mitigated if the underlying nutrigenomic weaknesses that are causing these changes are identified and supplemented nutritionally.

Methylation of cytosine is generally correlated with silencing of genes. One difference between bacterial and human genomes is that bacterial genes are *not* methylated at specific cytosine regions. **Research has shown that when mammalian genes are not methylated at these regions it can trick**

the immune system into reacting against itself and causing autoimmunity. New cell synthesis is needed in order for certain types of immune cells to expand and respond properly to an immune assault. These same immune cells are also involved in controlling the overall immune response, keeping it in balance. If there are Methylation Cycle problems or mutations, you may have trouble making the bases that are needed for new DNA synthesis. If you cannot make new DNA, then you cannot make these specialized immune cells and as a result you may lack immune system regulatory cells.

The immune system has the B cell "arm" that makes antibodies, known as humoral immunity and the T cell "arm" known as cellular immunity. If you are having trouble making new T cells, then the immune response may become more heavily weighted in the direction of B cells. The B cells have the ability to respond by making antibody, or auto antibody rather than making the range of T cells that regulate as well as fight infections. B cell clones expand and then are available for the future. So there is a somewhat greater need for new DNA synthesis for the T cell response than for the B cell response. Individuals with Methylation Cycle mutations are more at risk as they will have problems making regulatory T cells that help the body to control the B cells and prevent autoimmune antibodies. Auto antibodies can occur as a result of imbalances in immune regulation. If you are not making adequate T cells (methylation pathway mutations) then you may lack regulatory T cells and can end up with auto antibodies.

Methylation also plays a role in the ability of the immune system to recognize foreign bodies or antigens that it needs to respond to. Research has shown that methylation is decreased in humans with auto immune conditions. Impaired methylation of T cells may be involved in the production of auto antibodies. Studies from patients with systemic lupus erythrematosis (SLE) have shown that their T cells are undemethylated. **Impaired methylation of T cells may also be involved in the production of auto antibodies.** Studies from patients with systemic lupus erythrematosis (SLE) have shown that their T cells are undermethylated. As proper methylation function is restored, it should help in regaining immune function regulation. In several cases I have seen the level of auto antibodies decline after proper Methylation Cycle supplementation.

Methylation of DNA is also used to regulate immune cells. Immune receptor DNA is initially in the "OFF" state and is maintained that way until the immune cells need to differentiate. At that time the methyl groups are removed from the DNA in a highly regulated fashion.

Studies show that decreased methylation of cytosine regions in these immune genes may influence the balance of immune inflammatory cells known as TH1 and TH2. **The effect of methyl groups on the TH1/TH2 balance may be another mechanism by which decreased methylation may increase allergies.** There are two sets of T helper cells in the immune system, TH1 and TH2 cells. While TH1 cells are involved in cell mediated immune responses and toning down or regulating TH2 activity, the TH2 cells have been associated with humoral or B cell mediated responses and allergic responses. TH2 cells trigger the activation and recruitment of IgE antibody producing B cells, mast cells and eosinophils that are involved in allergic inflammation. In addition, when methylation is impaired it can lead to abnormally high levels of histamine. High levels of histamine are causative factors in allergic reactions. Optimal methylation function is needed to break down histamine so that it does not build up in the body, in addition to the effect of methylation on histamine levels.

The levels of various metabolites of the methylation pathway are important for protection from side effects of anesthesia. As early as 1942 it was recognized that the addition of methionine is preventative for side effects from the use of chloroform. Methionine affords protection from liver injury as a result of chloroform anesthesia. Methionine also protects against effects of nitrous oxide anesthesia. Nitrous oxide disrupts the activity of MTR, a central enzyme in the Methylation Cycle. Again, preloading with methionine appears to accelerate recovery and reduce side effects associated with this form of anesthesia. The neurological deterioration and death of an infant boy has been reported who had been anesthetized twice within a short time with the anesthetic nitrous oxide. Postmortem studies determined that this child had a deficiency of the MTHFR which is a principle enzyme in the Methylation Cycle.

The relationship between environmental toxins and DNA methylation is extremely complex. Environmental toxins can impact the extent to which DNA is methylated. *"A hypothesis that is gaining ground is that environmental factors achieve their effect by altering the epigenetic profile of the cell"* conversely epigenetics may *"thus explain why certain individuals are more susceptible to certain environmental toxins"* (Traynor, Neuron). **Furthermore, methylation is also required to clear environmental toxins from the body.** This process involves conjugating methyl groups to the toxins prior to removal. Most of the methyl groups that are used for detoxification are donated by SAMe. Elimination of inorganic arsenic from the body requires methylation. After methylation arsenic can be eliminated from the body in the urine. Differences in methylation may also account for susceptibility of different tissues to cadmium toxicity. In animal studies, methylation was necessary to induce metallothionein activity that was required for cadmium excretion. The methylation process is also the major means of detoxifying excess selenium in the body. Nutritional support for the methylation pathway was able to prevent strychnine induced seizures and death in animal models, as well as to be protective against carbon tetrachloride induced toxicity. Supplementation was also able to prevent ethanol induced decreases in Methylation Cycle function. Compounding the situation, environmental toxins are also able to have a negative impact on methylation. In experimental models, exposure of animals to environmental toxins during development appears to alter the pattern of DNA methylation. This change in DNA methylation is then maintained and carried forward to future generations of offspring. The heavy metals, arsenic, nickel and chromium are able to cause over methylation of DNA. This can result in turning "OFF" of important regulatory genes such as tumor suppressor genes. In addition, other environmental contaminants such as polycyclic aromatic hydrocarbons (PAH) and benzo(a)pyrene diol epoxide (BPDE) are able to bind to methylated cytosine regions of the DNA. Cadmium also inhibits the methylation of phospholipids, interfering with cellular membrane functions.

Undermethylation of the entire genome is referred to as global hypomethylation. Global hypomethylation when paired with over methylation of highly select repeated regions of the gene is associated with both aging and cancer.

Intermediates of the methylation pathway are known to decrease with age along with a decline in Methylation Cycle function. DNA methylation is also known to decrease with aging. Age related decreases in methylation can lead to decreased methylation of T cells which may in part explain changes in immune function with age. Age related decreases in methylation can result in increased levels of homocysteine, increasing the risk of arthritis, cancer depression and heart disease. This would suggest that increasing the body's level of methylation through supplementation may extend a healthy life span. Both undermethylation of tumor causing genes (no turn OFF) and overmethylation of tumor suppressing genes (turned OFF) have been well characterized as contributing factors to cancer.

Methylation is used to inactivate excess levels of endogenous products that may be harmful to the body. For instance, excess estrogen is inactivated by methylation, with SAMe donating a methyl group for this process. The inability to inactivate excess estrogen has been linked to an increased susceptibility to hormone sensitive cancers. Epidemiologic and mechanistic evidence suggests mutations in the Methylation Cycle are involved in colorectal neoplasia. Specifically, the role of certain MTHFR mutations, MTR and MTRR mutations have been implicated in colorectal cancer.

The overwhelming impact of Methylation Cycle mutations is exemplified by the article in Science News which reported that although identical twins have the identical DNA they often have differences in a number of traits including disease susceptibility. This study suggests that as twins go through life the environmental influences to which they are exposed affects which genes are actually turned on or off. Methyl groups can attach to the DNA in a similar way that charms attach to a charm bracelet. This modification of the DNA is what I have already described as epigenetic regulation. The combination of environmentally determined addition of these "charms" to the bracelet of DNA, combined with inherited DNA changes or mutations lead to an individual's susceptibility to disease. According to the scientist who headed this study, Dr. Manuel Estseller, *"My belief is that people are 50 percent genetics and 50 percent environment"*.

This statement should give us some understanding as to why mutations in the Methylation Cycle can be so devastating. Mutations in the Methylation Cycle affect the 50% that represents genetic susceptibility; this would be analogous to defects in the links of the chain of our charm bracelet. In addition, because methylation is also necessary for the epigenetic modification of the DNA, methylation also affects the environmental 50%.

Genes Commonly Methylated in Human Cancer and Their Role in Tumor Development

Role in Tumor Development	Site of Tumor
Deranged regulation of cell proliferation, cell migration, cell adhesion, cytoskeletal reorganization, and chromosomal stability	Breast, Lung, Esophageal
Implicated in DNA repair and transcription activation	Breast, Ovarian
Cyclin-dependent kinase inhibitor	GIT, Head and neck, NHL, Lung
Calcium/calmodulin-dependent enzyme that phosphorylates serine/threonine residues on proteins; Supression of apoptosis	Lung
Increasing proliferation, invasion, and/or metastasis	Breast, Thyroid, Gastric
Horomone resistance	Breast, Prostate
Loss of detoxification of active metabolites of several carcinogens	Prostate, Breast, Renal
Defective DNA mismatch repair and gene mutations	Colon, Gastric, Endometrium, Ovarian
p53-related gene involved in DNA repair and drug resistance	Lung, Brain
Unrestrained entry of cells into activation and proliferation	Leukemia, Lymphoma, Squamous cell carcinoma, Lung
Loss of negative regulator control of cell proliferation through inhibition of G_1/S-phase progression	Lung, Breast, Ovarian, Kidney, Nasopharyngeal
Failure to repress the transcription of cellular genes required for DNA replication and cell division	Retinoblastoma, Oligodendroglioma
Altered RNA stability through an erroneous degradation of RNA-bound proteins	Renal cell cancer

Das and Singal Journal Clinical Oncology, November 15, 2004 vol. 22 no. 22 4632-4642

If we take the analogy a step further to really understand the global impact of defects in this pathway we can view genetically inherited mutations in the methylation pathway as causing problems in the links of the bracelet and environmental effects creating a problem with the ability to put charms on the bracelet of DNA. **Problems in the Methylation Cycle therefore can affect 100% of our susceptibility to disease. This is why it is critical for health reasons to understand where our weaknesses in this pathway reside and then supplement appropriately to bypass these mutations.**

A second study that has also addressed the nature versus nurture question used animal models to look at this issue. Researchers were able to show that the adult response to stressful situations was heavily influenced by the interactions these same animals had as pups with their mothers at birth. Those pups with higher levels of care showed differences in the methylation patterns of stress related genes when compared with pups in the lower care test group. Dr. Szyf from the team at McGill University that conducted the study has stated that their study results *"…have bridged the gap, nurture is nature"*.

This work does suggest that the bridge between "nature and nurture" is the ability of nurturing to influence DNA methylation. However, nurture alone cannot be the answer. According to this study nurturing can influence epigenetic modification of DNA, so nurturing can affect the number of "charms on the bracelet". However if there are genetic mutations in the DNA sequence itself, the actual "links of the bracelet" this will also affect the overall methylation capacity in the body. **Without the mechanisms to produce the methyl groups, all of the nurturing in the world will not be able to overcome the lack in the production capacity for methylation.** In other words if the body cannot produce the charms for the bracelet it becomes a moot point how easily you are able to attach them to the bracelet. Nutrigenomic support to bypass these mutations is one mechanism to address the weaknesses in the DNA that would result in reduced capacity in this pathway.

CHAPTER 21

You Can Lead a Horse to Water

The Methylation Cycle that I have focused on in this book describes genetic weaknesses in the particular pathway that is involved in generating and utilizing methyl groups in the body. This central pathway is particularly amenable to nutrigenomic screening for genetic weaknesses. Defects in methylation lay the appropriate groundwork for the further assault of environmental and infectious agents and result in an increased risk for additional health conditions including diabetes, cardiovascular disease, thyroid dysfunction, neurological inflammation, chronic viral infection, neurotransmitter imbalances, atherosclerosis, cancer, aging, neural tube defects, Alzheimer's disease and autism. As a result of decreased activity in the Methylation Cycle due to mutations, there is a shortage of methyl groups in the body for a variety of important functions. Methyl groups are "CH3" groups that are moved around in the body to turn on or off genes. There are several particular sites in this pathway where blocks can occur as a result of genetic weaknesses. Supplementation with appropriate foods and nutrients can help bypass these mutations to allow for restored function of the pathway.

Because it's involved in so many processes, inefficient function or mutations along the methylation pathway can result in a wide range of conditions, including the following:

- Aging
- Allergic Reactions
- Alzheimer
- Anxiety
- Arthritis
- Autism
- Bowel dysfunction
- Cancer
- CFS/FM
- Chronic bacterial infections
- Chronic viral infections
- Cytoskeletal breakdown
- Down's syndrome
- Heart disease
- Herpes
- Huntington's disease
- Language and cognition impairment
- Leaky gut
- Leaky gut syndrome
- Metal toxicity
- Miscarraige
- Mitochondrial disease
- Neural tube defects
- Pneumonia
- Psoriasis
- Renal failure
- Rett's syndrome
- Schizophrenia
- Seizures
- Sleep disorders
- Systemic Lupus Erythematosus (SLE)
- Thyroid dysfunction

"*Methylation occurs a billion times a second throughout the body, affecting everything from fetal development to brain function. It regulates the expression of genes. It preserves the fatty membranes that insulate our cells. And it helps regulate the action of various hormones and neurotransmitters, including serotonin, melatonin, dopamine and adrenaline.* **Without methylation there could be no life as we know it**" (Cooney, Methyl Magic).

It has not been my desire to scare you, quite the contrary. **My goal is to empower you, to share information so that you have the knowledge and ability to bypass issues in this critical pathway so that you can chart your own personalized Roadmap to health.** By this point I would hope that you comprehend that this may be *the* pathway for a better, healthier existence. Now, it is up to you to change your stars, to chart a new path for your own health as well as the health of your future generations.

The discussion group is available at:
www.CH3Nutrigenomics.com

My Facebook page: **www.Facebook.com/DrAmyYasko**

My personal website: **www.DrAmyYasko.com**

Articles on Scribd: **www.Scribd.com/DrAmyYasko**

Additional resources including videos:
www.DrAmyYasko.com/Resources

Nutrigenomic analysis: **www.KnowYourGenetics.com**

CHAPTER 22

Spirituality and Our Unique DNA

Before my doctoral defense at Albany Medical College, my advisor suggested that I bring up the weak points in my thesis myself before they were pointed out by the committee. He suggested that I be direct and honest and make sure I was the one that identified and discussed the questionable data, not to wait to have someone else identify the problem areas. That was wonderful advice then and I still believe in being upfront, honest and noting where the weak points are rather than waiting to have someone else do it.

There have been two main complaints or criticisms of this program. The first, when I initially came out with this program the feedback was that it was too complicated. I have tried to rectify that situation by designing specially compounded supplements, by designing my own nutrigenomic test, by writing books and offering a workbook and answering questions online as well as giving presentations all to try to simplify and explain the program more thoroughly. This book is an even more basic introduction into the program for health and wellness based on balancing your Methylation Cycle. I feel that I have done my best to address that major criticism of the program.

The second area where I would say I have been misunderstood is with respect to my motivation. These criticisms come from those who do not know me, who have never spoken with me nor really delved into the program. I can understand how someone would question that I actually do put all of the information to implement this program online at no charge. I can see how that is hard to believe, but that is the truth. While you do have the option of ordering tests and supplements through Holistic Health International, that is not necessary in order to use this program. Only a small fraction of those using this program run tests for my comments or use the specially compounded supplements or tests I have designed. The magnitude of those using the program on their own, with their own doctors is quite overwhelming and frankly that is wonderful. If every person on the Facebook page or chat group wanted my personal feedback to implement the program I would need to stop offering that service. So, it is true, you can follow this program and have every bit of information about how to move forward on your Roadmap to Health by accessing the free online resources. You and your doctor can read the workbook, read the articles, watch the DVDs, look at the PPTs and read the transcripts that go along with the talks.

There is no fee. You can join the chat group and search for answers to questions and ask your own questions all at no cost. **So that gets us to why, why would I do this? Why would someone just share?**

The conventional wisdom is that it is not advised to talk about spirituality when it comes to science, as somehow the perception is that you cannot be a spiritual person and intrinsically rooted in science at the same time. But that is the reality. **I am a spiritual person who believes that if you are blessed in life with three healthy children who are beautiful inside and out, and a husband who supports you in every aspect of your life...that you pay it forward**. It has been a long time since I included a spiritual chapter in a book, as the common wisdom was that people will think differently of you if you openly share your thoughts and beliefs on the subject of spirituality. Well, some people will continue to disparage my motives regardless of what I say or do. Thus, I have chosen to end this book, designed to chart your Roadmap to health, on a spiritual note. I truly feel that just as herbs and supplements can help you to heal, so too can positive affirmations and spiritual intent make a difference in health and wellness.

I truly believe that our actions do matter, that we are here on this Earth to learn lessons and to change and grow as individuals in a positive manner. I take to heart the words of Lao Tzu: *"Watch your thoughts; they become words. Watch your words; they become actions. Watch your actions; they become habit. Watch your habits; they become character. Watch your character; it becomes your destiny".*

While our DNA is our biochemical destiny, we have the ability to improve that path with support for epigenetics and methylation. Our integrity and our spiritual destiny is a choice we make on a personal level. Yet these two seemingly disparate fields actually appear to be linked. There is more to our DNA than the bases that define our biochemical destiny and we can look to our DNA for its role in the mysteries of spirituality.

Dr. Craig Venter is a founder of one of the firms that led the Human Genome Project. He is quoted as remarking that, *"We have only 300 unique genes in the human genome that are not in the mouse. This tells me genes can't possibly explain all of what makes us what we are"*. This statement from an individual so intimately involved in the molecular biology and biotechnology of DNA sequences suggests that we need to look beyond the mere "spelling" of our DNA and RNA when it comes to our health.

Dr. Larry Dossey writes about three Eras of medicine that have progressed since the mid 19th century. According to Dr. Dossey *"Era I is good old everyday mechanical medicine, technical orthodox medicine. Drugs, surgery and radiation. Era I, which can be called "mechanical medicine" and which began roughly in the 1860s, reflects the prevailing view that health and illness are totally physical in nature, and thus all therapies should be physical ones, such as surgical procedures or drugs"* (Dossey, L, Reinventing Medicine, HarperCollins, 1999).

I simply describe Era I medicine as "if this, then that" medicine. This would include taking a specific herb to remedy a specific condition, a supplement to help balance a pathway or an antibiotic to eradicate a bacterial infection.

Era II medicine, according to Dr. Dossey, is how your mind affects your body. It acknowledges that stress and your frame of mind can have a negative impact on your body. It is what is commonly referred to as the Mind/Body connection.

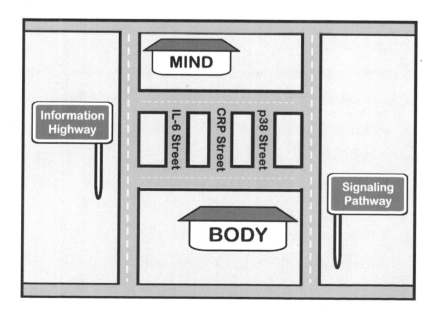

Very specific inflammatory mediators have been well characterized in terms of their ability to convey stress to the body. Mediators such as IL6, p38Map kinase and CRP are some of the information pathways that the mind uses to convert stress into harmful effects on the body. Scientific studies have reported that higher CRP levels were found in men in their 70's with less social interaction as compared with men with more social interaction. Elevated CRP is associated with levels of inflammation and is a risk factor for a number of inflammatory disorders including heart disease, colon cancer and Alzheimer's disease among others. A study published in the very prestigious journal Proceedings of the National Academy of Science reported that after following individuals over a six year time period, increases in IL6 have been correlated with stress. A series of papers in this same journal, underscored the relationship between stress and yet another inflammatory mediator, p38MAP kinase. These types of relationships between well-defined concrete, measurable inflammatory mediators and the ability of the mind to trigger the release of these mediators falls under the domain of Era II medicine. Keeping that "in mind" you should never underestimate the power of spirituality or positive thoughts and the impact it can have on your health.

Patients with osteoarthritis who believed in their ability to perform tasks were less debilitated after 3 years than those who were less confident (Loucks, Bottom Line Health).   Conversely, research from

McGill University (Spirituality and Health) has shown that brains from senior citizens with low self-esteem had atrophied leading to a higher incidence of memory loss than those who felt good about themselves. People scoring higher on anxiety tests were 25% more likely to have premalignancies (Clinical Pearls). Two separate studies support a correlation between prayer and the ability to become pregnant (Cuvelier, Psychology Today). Your frame of mind, as evidenced by your spirituality, appears to increase life span (Bottom Line Health).

This mind/body effect can be very powerful even when it comes to surgery. In a study involving 30 patients, only 12 received the actual surgical treatment; the other 18 only received a sham surgical procedure. Neither the participants, nor the medical attending staff knew which procedure each participant received. One year later, the 10 patients who *thought* they received the transplant reported better physical, emotional, and social functioning than the 20 who believed they had received the sham surgery. The medical staff also reported improved outcomes in the patients who believed they had received the treatment. Of the 10 who were doing better, and believed they had received the actual surgical procedure, only 4 of them had in fact received the treatment. This study helps to confirm that believing in a treatment and the power of positive thinking help to make it more effective (McRae, Arch Gen Psychiatry).

"Era II began to take shape in the period following World War II. Physicians began to realize, based on scientific evidence, that disease has a "psychosomatic" aspect: that emotions and feelings can influence the body's functions. Psychological stress, for example, can contribute to high blood pressure, heart attacks, and ulcers. This was a radical advance over Era I. Era II is involved any time we talk about mind/body events within the person. My mind affecting my brain affecting my body, for good or ill. It's confined to the present moment, it's "here and now "medicine, it's local" (Dossey, L. Reinventing Medicine).

Era III medicine is how "my" mind affects "your" body. This is an area that is not completely understood; yet the power of belief or prayer and its effect on healing has been proven to occur. *"Era III is mind/body medicine with a different slant. The recently developing Era III goes even further by proposing that consciousness is not confined to one's individual body. Nonlocal mind – mind that is boundless and unlimited - is the hallmark of Era III. An individual's mind may affect not just his or her body, but the body of another person at a distance, even when that distant individual is unaware of the effort. You can think of Era II as illustrating the personal effects of consciousness and Era III as illustrating the transpersonal effects of the mind. It's important to remember that these eras are not mutually exclusive; rather they coexist, overlap, and are used together, as when drugs are used with psychotherapy, and surgery is used with prayer"* (Dossey, L.

Reinventing Medicine).

We do know from studies being conducted around the world that there are hard facts and statistics that support the idea that Era III medicine is a reality. Studies at the Princeton Engineering Anomalies Research Laboratory have been conducted for over a decade by the ex-Dean of Engineering Dr. Robert Jahn and his colleague Brenda Dunne. In their remote-sensing experiments, the scientists had one person in Princeton attempting to mentally send a computer-selected image to a person 6000 miles away. Significantly, the receiver was able to get the message in great detail. This is mind operating outside of our conventional views of space and time.

Similar instances of distance communication are seen in nature. *"When a queen ant is spatially separated from her colony, building still continues fervently and according to plan. If the queen is killed, however, all work in the colony stops. No ant knows what to do. Apparently the queen sends the building plans"* also from far away via the group consciousness of her subjects. *She can be as far away as she wants, as long as she is alive. In man hyper communication is most often encountered when one suddenly gains access to information that is outside one's knowledge base"* (Fosar, G. and Bludorf, F., Vernetzte Intelligenz).

So too, we know that distant prayer, or if you prefer positive thoughts or affirmations, have been shown to affect a number of health conditions. Research at Duke University Medical Center in Durham, North Carolina studied the effects of prayer on patients undergoing cardiac procedures such as catheterization and angioplasty. Patients receiving prayer had up to 100% fewer side effects from these procedures than people not prayed for (Archives of Internal Med., Krucoff, American Heart Journal, Grunberg, Cardiology Rev). A recent article from the ordinarily "very Era I medical journal", the Journal of the American Medical Association, noted that seeing a loved one in pain activates some of the same brain areas that are mobilized when we experience pain ourselves; a case of *my* mind reacting to *your* body (Journal American Medical Association).

One would need a guide to navigate uncharted areas through the African rainforest as it would be impossible to get to your destination without that guide who is familiar with the territory. Similarly, just because we don't know the way to get there, does not mean that a place does not exist. In terms of Era III medicine we do not have to know exactly which roads to transverse to arrive at the final destination, just simply to acknowledge that the destination and the roads do exist. For some it is a place they would prefer not to even attempt to travel to, and we must respect that choice.

The point is that seemingly unconventional pathways do exist even if we do not yet know what they are or we do not fully understand them. It is sufficient to be open-minded and be aware that they may in fact have an impact on our health.

For those who are skeptics it should be intriguing to now learn that only 2% to 5% of the genome encodes protein. In other words as far as we know at this time, only 5% of the DNA in each of our cells, that same DNA that is long enough to stretch all the way to the sun and back again, is used for anything that we would consider useful. Among the 5% that is actually used there is a high degree of similarity between diverse species. An in depth analysis of the conservation of genes between species suggests "...*the existence of a selective force in the overall design of genetic pathways to maintain a highly connected class of genes*" (Stuart, J. Science).

As described in the article "So Much Junk DNA In Our Genome" (Ono, S. Brookhaven Symp Biol) approximately 95% of our DNA is not utilized to make proteins and hence must be "junk". However, recent work has shown that this so called "junk" DNA is more highly conserved between species than the other 5% that is used to make proteins. The high degree of conservation between species of this other 95% suggests that there is an important function to these regions that has not yet been determined (Dermitzakis, E. et al, Science).

Former senior computer systems designer, now turned author, Gregg Braden demonstrates in his book The God Code, that *"When correlated with an ancient alphabet, the code of all life becomes a translatable message in our cells"* (Braden, G., The God Code).

The role that our DNA may play in communication is confirmed by recent discoveries involving dolphins. *"Beyond being life's blueprint, DNA plays a powerful role in newly discovered communications between dolphins and humans, according to a team of Cetacean (dolphin and whale) researchers at the Sirius Institute on the Big Island of Hawaii. An ongoing study there shows these marine mammals receive and transmit sound signals capable of affecting the genetic double helix...using natural biotechnology DNA is activated, new research shows, by waves and particles of energized sound and light which, more than chemicals or drugs, switch genes "on" or "off"* (Tetrahedron).

Russian scientists have taken this premise a step further. Scientists in the fields of biophysics and molecular biology have collaborated with linguists and geneticists to study this 95% "junk DNA". The results of their work suggest that DNA is not only responsible for the physical construction of the body but that it also serves as one huge data storage and communication system. The Russian linguists found that this highly conserved 95% of DNA that was apparently useless followed the same rules as all human language.

"To this end they compared the rules of syntax (the way in which words are put together to form phrases and sentences), semantics (the study of meaning in language forms) and the basic rules of grammar. They found that the alkalines of our DNA follow a regular grammar and do have set rules just like our languages" (Fosar, G. and Bludorf, F., Vernetzte Intelligenz). The results of this work may help to explain aspects of Era III medicine as well as certain facets of clairvoyance, intuition as well as spontaneous and remote acts of healing.

This 95% to 98% "junk DNA" that is not utilized to make protein is a situation that may be unique to certain species. Bacteria, for instance, use the majority of their DNA for protein production. This has led to the suggestion that the function of the majority of human DNA is to make RNAs that may be involved in communication and cellular regulation. *"Less than 2% of the 3.2 billion bases in the human genome code for proteins...Does this suggest that the reason for the 'superiority' of humans lies in the 98% of the genome that does not code for proteins? Is it not conceivable that the end products of many mammalian genes are not proteins, but RNAs?...Is it conceivable that certain RNA molecules are the actual creators and controllers of life?"* (Pieztch, J. Understanding the RNAissance).

And so we have come full circle. Whether we quote Dr. Gary Zweiger, geneticist from Stanford and Columbia Universities, Genentech, Incyte and Agilent Technologies, *"Genes are the most obvious conveyors of information with living beings... As information it does not really matter how the gene is encoded, so long as the message can be received and decoded... Molecular messages may move a bit slower than the speed of light, but as information they are essentially no different than messages sent over phone lines or reflected off of satellites: they all may be transduced, digitized and stored"*. Or we may quote the Russian scientists: *"DNA...also serves as data storage and in communication. Living chromosomes function ... like computers"*. Regardless of whom we quote we come to the same conclusion. We can take advantage of this inherent information within our genes and be cognizant of the imbalances in these pathways in order to personalize our nutritional support and optimize our overall health and well-being.

About the Author

"The inclination to goodness is imprinted deeply in the nature of man. It is our uniqueness as a species, coupled with our fundamental character of goodness that opens the door for the message in our cells to see real and lasting change in our lives." (Braden, G. The God Code, Hay House Publishers, 2004)

Dr. Yasko lives in a rural town in western Maine with her husband of over 25 years, her three daughters and two Newfoundland dogs. She holds a doctorate in microbiology, immunology, and infectious diseases with an award for

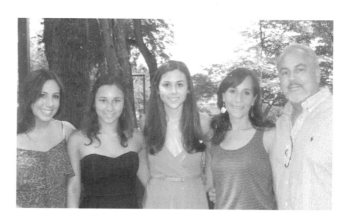

outstanding academic excellence from Albany Medical College.

Dr. Yasko completed two research fellowships at Strong Memorial hospital in Rochester NY; one as a member of the Dept. of Pediatrics and Infectious Diseases, the other as a member of the Wilmont Cancer Center. Her third fellowship was in Cell Biology in the Department of Hematology at Yale Medical Center in New Haven prior to joining a biotechnology company in Connecticut.

Dr. Yasko later co-founded a successful biotechnology company, where she was recognized as an expert in the field of DNA/RNA based diagnostics and therapeutics. Prior to shifting her focus to integrative healthcare she was consultant to the medical, pharmaceutical, and research communities for almost 20 years with an expertise in biochemistry, molecular biology, and biotechnology. Dr. Yasko continued her education in the area of integrative healthcare, receiving two additional degrees, a Doctor of Naturopathy and a Doctor of Natural health. She is also a Fellow of the American Association of Integrative Medicine.

Amy Yasko
Ph.D., NHD, AMD, HHP, FAAIM

Degrees/Certification

- Doctorate Microbiology/Immunology/Infectious Disease
- Certified Alternative Medical Practitioner
- Certified Holistic Health Practitioner
- Fellow-American Association Integrative Medicine
- College of Physicians-Certified Diplomat
- College of Herbal Medicine-Certified Diplomat
- College of Pharmaceutical Sciences-Certified Diplomat

Education

Albany Medical College of Union University

- Dept. Microbiology/Immunology & Infectious Disease; Ph.D. - graduated Summa Cum Laude
- Research - Antibiotic Resistance and Transport; Dean's Award for Research Excellence
- Cytochromes and Antibiotic Resistance

Clayton College of Natural Health

- Doctor Naturopathy; Graduated with Highest Honors
- NHD – Doctor Natural Health; Graduated with Highest honors

Colgate University

- Double Major - Chemistry and Fine Arts
- B.A. - Graduated Magna Cum Laude

Academic Positions

- Yale Medical Center
  Department of Hematology
  New Haven, Connecticut
  Fellow - Eukaryotic/Prokaryotic Shuttle Vectors

- Strong Memorial Hospital
  Cancer Center
  Rochester, New York
  Fellow – Mammalian Retroviruses

- Strong Memorial Hospital
  Dept. Pediatrics & Infectious Disease
  Rochester, New York
  Fellow – Bacterial Vaccines

Industrial Positions

Neurological Research Institue, LLC.
 Consultant
 Complementary & Alternative Health Care

Holistic Health International, LLC.
 Scientific Consultant
 Complementary & Alternative Health Care
Oligos Etc. Inc.
 Cofounder and Vice President
 Synthesis and Development of Nucleic Acid based drugs
 As anti-microbial and anti-inflammatory agents
Biotix Inc.
 Cofounder and Vice President
 Development of automated DNA Synthesizer

International Biotechnologies Inc. (now Kodak/IBI)
 Director of Research and Development
 Development of Molecular Biology Kits

Honors and Associations

2004 CASD Award for RNA Research in Autism
Who's Who in the World
Who's Who in American Women
Who's Who in Science and Engineering
Who's Who in Young Professionals
Who's Who in Emerging Leaders
Scientific Advisory Board-National Foundation Alternative Medicine (NFAM)
American College for Advancement in Medicine
Founding Member of National Integrative Medicine Council (NIMC)
American Naturopathic Medical Association
Society for Neuroscience
American Nutraceutical Association
Association of Drugless Practitioners
National Center for Homeopathy
American Association of Pharmaceutical Scientists
Marion Foundation
Association of Medical Diagnostics Manufacturers
American Chemical Society – Division of Medicinal Chemistry
American Society for Microbiology
Life Extension Foundation
New York Biotechnology Association
New York Academy of Sciences
American Association for the Advancement of Science
National Association of Female Executives
Sigma XI Research Society

Publications, Interviews & Presentations

1. Yasko, A. (2014) Roadmap to Health in Autism: What the Experts Know Resource Booklet, 4th edition.

1. Yasko, A. (2014) Feel Good Nutrigenomics. Neurological Research Institute, Bethel Maine

2. Yasko, Amy. (2013) Interview with Eva Herr. Infinite Consciousness.1 September 2013.

3. Yasko, A. (2013). Simplified Roadmap to Health.

4. Yasko, A.(2013) Methylation, Genetics and Diagnostics in Diagnostic Testing and Functional Medicine by Ameer Rosic.

5. Mullan, N. and A.Yasko. (2013). Aluminum Toxicity in Mitochondrial Dysfunction and ASD. Autism Science Digest, Issue 05.

6. Yasko, A. (2013) Using Nutrigenomics to Optimize Supplement Choices in Cutting Edge Therapies for Autism by Siri and Lyons. Chapter 20.

7. Yasko, A. (2012) NRI Autism Conference, Portland, ME

8. Yasko, A and N.Mullan. (2012). Gastrointestinal Balance and Neurotransmitter Formation. Autism Science Digest, Issue 04 July.

9. Mullan, N and A. Yasko (2012). Demystifying Genes: Your Child's Most Important Biochemistry. Autism Science Digest, Issue 03.

10. Yasko, A. (2011) NRI Autism Conference, Los Angeles, CA

11. Mullan, N and A.Yasko (2011) Methionine and Methylation: Chicken or the Egg. Autism Science Digest. Issue 1 April.

12. Yasko, A. (2011) Role of H.Pylori in Autism & Professional Training Session at AutismOne Chicago, IL

13. Yasko, A. and N.Mullan (2010). How Bacterial Imbalances May Predispose to Seizure Disorder. Autism File. Issue 38

14. Yasko, A. (2010) NRI Autism Conference, Boston, MA

15. Yasko, Amy. (2010) Interview with Eva Herr. Infinite Consciousness.14 February 2010.

16. Yasko, A. (2009) Autism: Pathways to Recovery. Neurological Research Institute, Bethel Maine

17. Yasko, A (2009) Assessment of Metals & Microbes in Autism & Professional Training Session Autism One Conference, Chicago, IL

18. Yasko, A. (2008) Interview with Jill Neimark in Curing the Children of Silent Spring. Spirituality and Health January 2008.

19. Yasko A. (2008) Individualized Approach to Autism lecture at AutismOne Chicago

20. Yasko, A (2007) Interviewee with Jill Neimark in Autism: It's Not Just in the Head. Discover Magazine March 2007.

21. Yasko, A. (2006) Interviewee, Autism Film Premier, Finding the Words San Francisco CA

22. Yasko, A. (2006) Beyond Autism Conference Boston MA

23. Yasko, Amy. (2006) Interview with Teri Small. Autism: Help, Hope, and Healing. Autism One Radio. IL. 25 July 2006, 1 Aug. 2006.

24. Yasko, Amy. (2006) Interview with Burton Goldberg. Do No Harm.

25. Yasko, A. (2006) A Comprehensive Analysis of Autism: From Metals to Mutations Conference Phoenix AZ

26. Yasko, A. and G. Gordon (2006) Nutrigenomic Testing and the Methylation Pathway. Townsend Newsletter. 270: 69.

27. Yasko, A. and G. Gordon (2006) The Puzzle of Autism. Revised Ed. Matrix Press.

28. Yasko, A. (2005) Genetic Bypass: Using Nutriton to Bypass Genetic Mutations. Matrix Publishing NY, NY.

29. Yasko, A. (2005) The Role of RNA in Addressing Multifactorial Disease. Annals Fourth Stromboli Conference on Aging and Cancer.

30. Yasko, A (2005) Speaker, ACAM Alternative Medical Conference Anaheim, CA

31. Yasko, A (2005) Speaker, NDHM Autism Conference Scottsdale, AZ

32. Yasko, A. (2005) Speaker, Stromboli Conference Cancer/Antiaging Stromboli, Italy

33. Yasko, A. and G. Gordon (2005) A Mutifactorial Approach to Heart Disease. Townsend Newsletter, May 2005.

34. Yasko, Amy. (2005) Interview with Deborah Ray. The Deborah Ray Show. Healthy Talk Radio. FL. 12 May 2005.

35. Yasko, Amy. (2005) Interview with Dr. Majid Ali. Science, Health, Healing. WBAI, NY. 9 May 2005.

36. Yasko, A. (2005) Speaker, ACAM, Alternative Medical Conference Orlando, FL

37. Yasko, Amy. (2005) Interview with Dr. Dennis Courtney. AM Impact on Your Health. WKHB, PA. 21 Mar. 2005, 23 Mar. 2005, 30 Mar. 2005.

38. Yasko, Amy. (2005) Interview with Burton Goldberg. Health News. WBAI, NY. 2 Mar. 2005.

39. Yasko, Amy. Interview with Elizabeth Nelson. Finding the Words. 2005. PBS.

40. Yasko, A. (2004) Speaker, CASD Autism Conference Austin, TX

41. Yasko, A. and G. Gordon (2004) Heal Your Body Naturally. Explore 13(6).

42. Gordon, G. and A. Yasko (2004) A Unique Approach to Metal Detoxification. Explore 13(5).

43. Gordon, G. and A. Yasko (2004) RNA Based Therapies in Nutritional Medicine. Explore 13(2).

44. Yasko, A. (2003).Speaker, New Dimensions in Medicine & Health. Phoenix, AZ

45. Yasko, A. (2003) Autism: An Approach to Reversing the Process.

46. Yasko, A. (2003) Neurological Inflammation: An Approach to Reversing the Process.

47. Yasko, A. (2002) Speaker, NFAM, Alternative Medical Conference Washington , DC

48. Yasko, A. (2002) Role of Excitotoxins in Autistic Type Behavior.

49. Bates, Reddoch, Hansakul, Arrow(Yasko), Dale, Miller. (2002) Biosensor detection of triplex formation by modified oligonucleotides. Anal Biochem. 15; 307(2):235-43.

50. Dale, RMK, Amy Arrow (Yasko), Woolf, Thompson, Gatton. (1996) On the Quality Control of Antisense Oligonucleotides. Antisense and Nucleic Acid Drug Development. 6 (3):151.

51. Dale, RMK Amy Arrow (Yasko), Terry Thompson. Oligonucleotide- Containing Pharmacological Compositions and Their Use. US Patent number: 8188259, Patent number: 8183361

52. Dale, RMK, Amy Arrow (Yasko), Steve Gatton, Terry Thompson. Protonated/acidified nucleic acids and methods of use. US Patent number: 6211349

53. Dale, RMK, Steve Gatton, Amy Arrow (Yasko), A. Pulmonary delivery of protonated/acidified nucleic acids. Patent number: 6211162

54. Dale, RMK, Gatton, Arrow (Yasko), A. Devices for Improved Wound Management. Patent number: 8435960, Patent number: 6627215

55. Arrow (Yasko), A., Dale, Thompson. Therapeutic Antisense Phosphodiesterase Inhibitors. US Patent Application number: 20030045490

56. Woolf, Tod, Amy Arrow (Yasko), RMK Dale. Three Component Chimeric Antisense Oligonucleotides. US Patent number: 7691996, Patent number: 6958239

57. Arrow (Yasko), A. RMK Dale, S. Raza, S. Srivastava. Oligonucleotide phosphate esters. US Patent number: 6015886

58. Arrow (Yasko), A., S.Gatton, RMK Dale, T. Thompson. Antimicrobial Compounds and their use. US Patent number: 7176191

59. Dale, RMK and Amy Arrow (Yasko). (1989) A rapid single stranded cloning sequencing, insertion, and deletion strategy. Recombinant DNA Methodology, p.711 Editors: Wu. Grossman, Moldave. Academic Press, NY.

60. Henderson, M., Arrow (Yasko), A. Dale, RMK. (1989) Rapid Synthesis, cleavage, and deprotection of DNA sequencing primers. American Biotechnology Laboratory 7 (3): 20.

61. Henderson, M., Arrow (Yasko), A., Dale, RMK. (1989) Chemical integrity and biological activity of synthetic DNA. American Biotechnology Laboratory 7 (6):22.

62. Dale, RMK and Amy Arrow (Yasko). (1987) A rapid single stranded cloning sequencing, insertion and deletion strategy. In: Methods in Enzymology 204:155.

63. Arrow (Yasko), A., P. Miller, J. Mueller, and H. Taber (1987) Bacterial uptake of Aminoglycoside Antibiotics. Microbiological Reviews 51:439-457.

64. Arrow (Yasko), A. and H. Taber (1986) Streptomycin accumulation by Bacillus subtils requires both a membrane potential and cytochrome aa33. Antimicrobial Agents Chemotherapy 29: 143-148.

65. Faletto, D.L., A. Arrow (Yasko) and I.G. Macara (1985) A very Early Decrease in Phosphatidylinositol Turnover Precedes the Decrease in c-myc Expression Accompanying Induction of Friend Erythroleukemia Cell Differentiation. Cell, 43:315.

Appendix

Yasko Methylation Pathway

1. The four cycles that make up the Methylation Cycle. This first diagram shows the pathways and the biochemical compounds that are a part of these cycles.

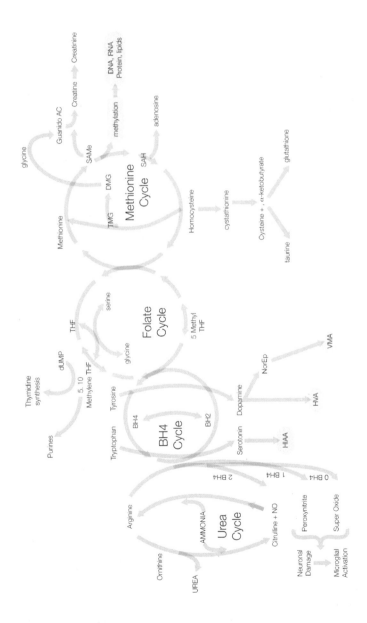

Yasko Methylation Pathway

2 The second diagram layers on the location of the genes in the nutrigenomic test to show where the possible locations of SNPs are in these biochemical pathways. The location of the where these genes act on these pathways are in color.

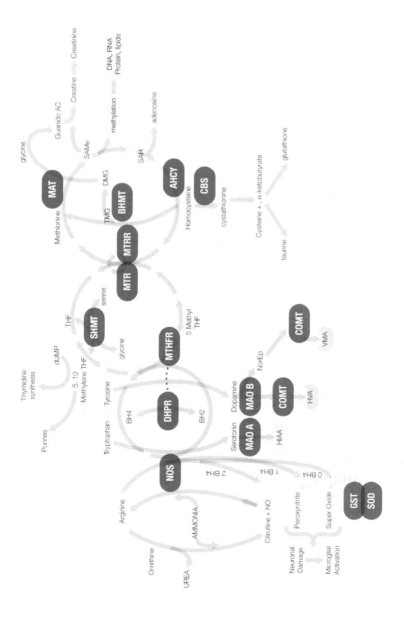

Yasko Methylation Pathway

3 The products of the genes often require what are called "cofactors" which are helpers that aid the gene in their function. The cofactors are noted in purple circles.

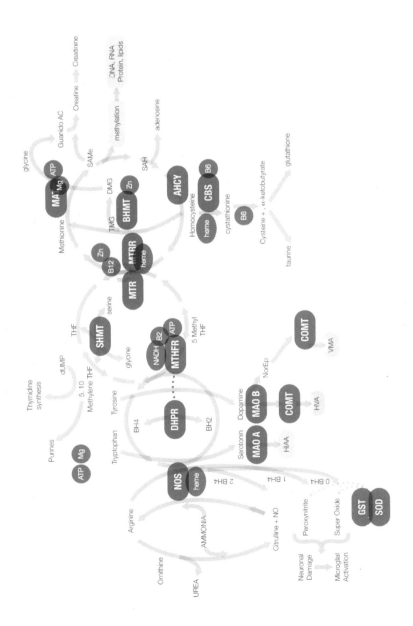

Yasko Methylation Pathway

4 There are places where nutritional support can be added to feed into these pathways. This helps to get around blocks due to malfunctions in the blue boxed genes. The places and names of the supplements that can be added to bypass mutations and where they can feed in to help with these pathways are in green.

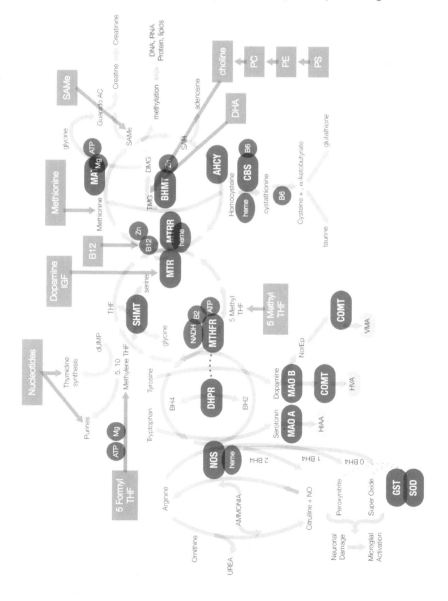

Yasko Methylation Pathway

5   Toxic metals can inhibit steps in these pathways even if there are not blocks due to mutations. Also products from the pathway can inhibit other reactions in the pathway. The locations of where the pathways are inhibited are noted in red.

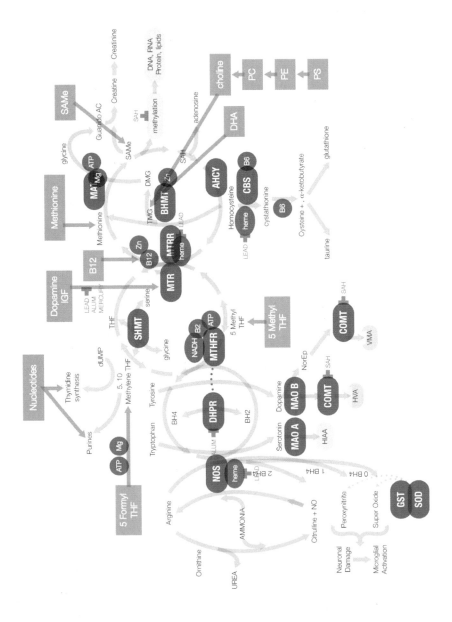

Yasko Methylation Pathway

© Content and diagrams may not be reproduced without express permission from NRI

6   The actual SNPs, or mutations in the genes are noted in pink.
    Recall that the genes in this pathway that are looked at by
    nutrigenomic testing are in blue boxes. The pink boxes show
    where the mutations in these genes occur thus affecting the
    position in the cycle where they are located.

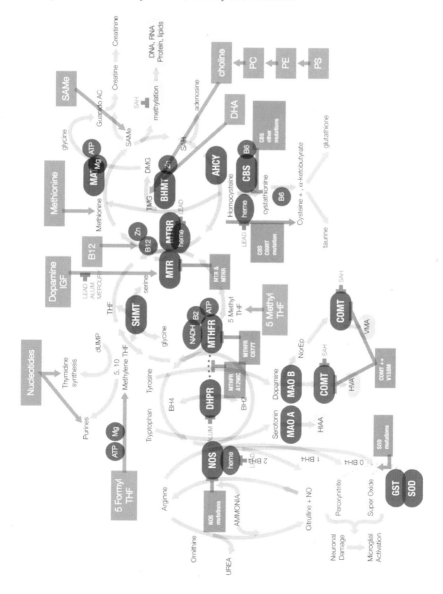